"International Breakthrough In Neuroscience In 2017"

Neuroscience of
Mind Empowerment and
Metacognition

Prof. Anees Akhtar
Co author: Prof. Dr Nasim Khan

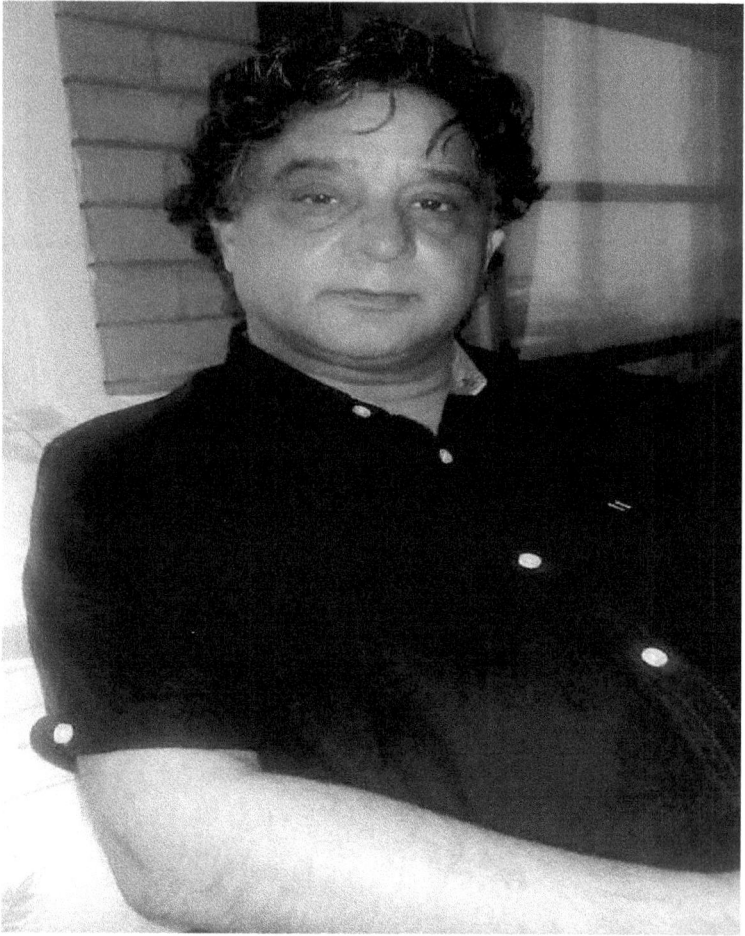

Neurocosmic Brain

Neuroscience of Mind Empowerment and Metacognition

Epigenetics, Neuroplasticity, Meditation, and Music Therapy

Prof. Anees Akhtar and Dr Nasim Khan

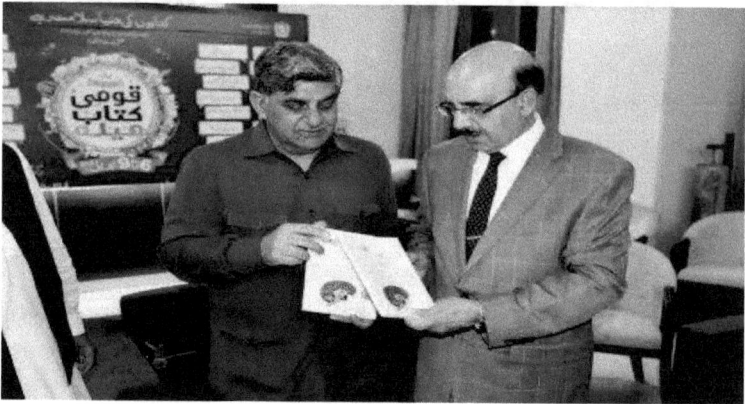

Co-Author Dr. Nasim Khan presenting the book to the President of Azad Jammu And Kashmir at the National Book Festival Islamabad, Pakistan.

"The authors passionately believe there is no way to achieve societal or national growth and prosperity other than by making the brains of nations more conscious, smarter, functional and advanced by the theory of Mind Empowerment and its Neuro-cosmic Ideology."

Dedicated to our late parents and sister. Anees extends heartfelt thanks to his supportive and loving wife.

Table Of Contents

Prologue

The majestic power of words and ideas in this book fulfil Nikola Tesla's exultant statement:

"I do not think there is any thrill that can go through the human heart, like that felt by the inventor as he sees some creation of the brain unfolding to success". **Nikola Tesla.**

"It is the sign of a good book when the book reads you". **Søren Kierkegaard.**

Embrace this book as it is privileged to have a breakthrough in the field of *'Mind Sciences'* — an innovation in the self-support industry, winning 'Multiple International Awards' in 2018 - 2019:

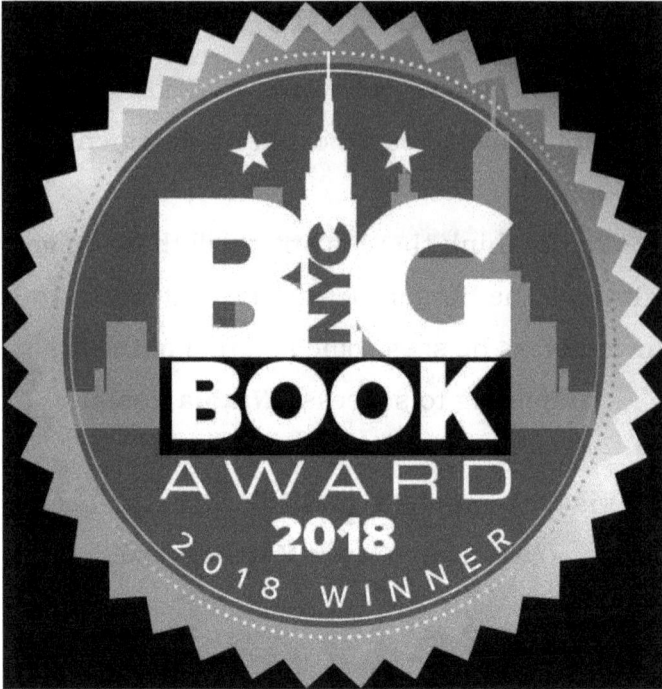

1.   NYC Big Book Award.

2.   Book Excellence Award.

3.   Independent Press Award.

It presents efficacious messages and energy in its words, innovative thoughts and ideas that have the ability to empower and heal a dysfunctional mind and transform you into a prosperous, healthy, blissful, super-functional being. It also has therapeutic support for minds with neurodegenerative diseases.

The strategy of goal setting, applied with strong healing, inspirational and epitomising effects of *Music Therapy and Meditation* will reinforce human epigenetics and positively alter human DNA and its gene expression. With optimistic and positive thoughts, you can rebuild your genetics and body according to the determination, goals and aims of your life.

Consequently, instead of living a life at the mercy of your *predisposed genetic makeup* for many illnesses, social and mental misfortunes, as well as negative thoughts, you can live a life of health, wealth, and happiness. Feeding your mind with positive thoughts, attitudes, humble gratitude of rewarding virtue encompassed within the energy of healing synchronisation of your mind – that has 1000 Terabytes of memory-holding capacity – you will make your brain a powerful mind-magnet, attracting an ample amount of positive healing energy to start a healthy chain reaction of new therapeutic chemicals in your body and mind.

These will not be like your previous negative reactions that were harming your mind and body's physiology and anatomy. As soon as you start channelling new energy into your body through positive thoughts, emotions and feelings, you will be less prone to *predisposed genetic makeup* for misery and misfortune.

Now, you are tapping new strategies for overcoming negative behaviour and attitude, which is already affecting your DNA and gene expression and is beginning to suppress many lethal genes that were predisposed to trigger illnesses like Cancer, Diabetes, Cardiovascular Diseases, Schizophrenia, and numerous Neurodegenerative Diseases like Alzheimer's, Parkinson's, Huntington's as well as Dyslexia, Autism and Depression.

Now, as you are in the process to improve your fate and fortune, you need to follow the rules and disciplines of the *'Neuroscience of Mind Empowerment and Metacognition'*. This book, with its *Models of Abundance*, prepares you to achieve high aims and goals to acquire a thriving, vigorous, affluent and prosperous life with a positive attitude by:

1. Art of Creativity and Intuition.
2. Goal Setting.
3. Epigenetics and Neuroplasticity.
4. Meditation and Music Therapy.

The effective strategies of this book's model of 'Mind Empowerment', awarded numerous accolades, have been carefully reviewed and justified by many experts in this field. Successful input of this effective software-like model of 'Mind Empowerment' in your 'soft-wired mind' will give you a substantial output and impact in your life in the form of abundance, health, and happiness.

Ultimately, you could monitor the positive effects of this *neuroplasticity* in your mind via MRI scans of your brain in clinical settings. As a virtue of your willpower and positive attitude, you *will* experience gradual changes in the anatomy and physiology of your mind. Spiritually and psychologically, you will feel integrated with your community, culture and ideology.

Acknowledgement

The development of this book has been the most stimulating journey and learning experience for both myself, Prof. Anees Akhtar, and Prof. Nasim Khan. We would like to express our gratitude to our brothers and sisters for this support in helping us complete this manuscript. Our heartiest regards to Dr. A. Q. Khan (world-renowned scientist), for participating as Chief Guest in the inaugural ceremony of our book at the International Islamic University. We are also thankful to Dr. Masoom Yasin Zai (Rector IIUI Islamabad), for his well-equipped venue that helped us host the book-launching ceremony and to Dr. Khaleeq Uz Zaman (Neurosurgeon) for participating as a Neuroscience expert and speaker.

We are highly grateful to NBF Pakistan's M.D., Dr. Inam ul Haq Javaid (M.D. NBF), for his kind invitation to Prof. Anees Akhtar as an overseas Book Ambassador 2018-19 at the Pakistan Annual National Book Fair that was hosted in Islamabad.

We greatly regard Dr. Tufail Hussain Tahir (Surgeon and Assistant Professor Poonch Medical College Rawlakot), Dr. Mehmood Khan (D.G. Health, Sate of A.J. & K. (Rtd.) Chairman, Red Crescent (Rtd.), Professor Dr. Mahroof Tahir (St. Cloud State University USA) for their assistance and consecutive inspiration in the development of our 'Mind Empowerment Theory'.

We are deeply grateful to M. Abbas Ali Khan, Nottingham (Late) for his consistent motivation and keen interest in the development of our lifelong learning, research, writing and speaking skills.

We are also indebted to the following friends and colleagues who have shown exuberant interest and inspiration in the creation of this book.

We greatly regard Professor Dr. Sarfraz Khan, Prof. Naseer Khan and Dr. Faisal, for facilitating us with opportunities to host seminars and workshops in their faculties and departments to enable us to share our valuable knowledge with their academic staff and research students. We extend our heartiest thanks to Prof. Imtiaz, Prof. Khalid, Prof. Dr. Saghir Khan, Principal Post Graduate College Rawlakot.

We also extend our gratitude to Dr. Awais Chaudhary. I extend special thanks to Dr. Alan Hargreaves, Dr. Adrian Slater, Prof. Richard Jenkins, Dr. Mark Fowler, Dr. Sandra Kirk, Dr. Shamim Ahmad, Prof. Stephen Forsythe and Dr. David Hughes, who have transmitted exclusive scientific ideas and innovations in Biotechnology and Biomedical Science.

We are grateful to Nottingham Speakers' Club (England) president Alan Young, ex-president Mr. Martin Cox, and Mr. Dennis Apple, in extending opportunities to speak in club meetings; we also appreciate Mr. Scott Warren for extending invitations to talk in the Nottingham Philosophy Club (England) meetings. We honour the efforts of our copy editors for their editing, transcribing and proofreading. Our grateful thanks go to all the staff of Seo-Prohub UK and especially the consultants Anthony Wills for their hard work in preparing the manuscript of the book for publishing.

We are very grateful to Dr. Syed Naheem Jafari (Calgary, Canada), renowned Virologist, Vaccinologist, Popular Intellectual and Enlightened Spiritual, and to Dr. Syed Naveed Imam (Founder of Brain Microchip) (Sitar-e-Imtiaz, Pakistan) Head of Cell Biology, University of Calgary, Hotchkiss Brain Institute for joining our "Neurocosmic Brain Research Project" to collaborate for future publications and innovations.

Introduction

The human Mind is the most powerful thing in the Universe. *'Mind Empowerment Science'* is the powerful methodology that enables us to harness all aspects of knowledge and wisdom to achieve success, wellbeing, fortune and pleasure from the Universe. We can harness the mental ability of history's greatest thinkers, artists and scientists, to allow their influence to expand our minds and create universal beauty and goodness in the world. For instance:

Philosophy: Aristotle, Frederick Engels, Georg Hegel. Karl Marx and Plato.

Science: Marie Curie, Thomas Edison, Albert Einstein, Galileo Galilei, Isaac Newton, Louis Pasteur, Orville and Wilbur Wright.

Art: Michelangelo, Raphael, Rembrandt and Leonardo da Vinci.

Literature: Charles Dickens, Faiz Ahmed Faiz, Allama Iqbal, Victor Hugo, Habib Jalib, John Keats, John Milton, William Shakespeare and Percy Bysshe Shelley.

Psychology: Sigmund Freud, William James, Karl

Jung and Jean Piaget.

Music: Ludwig van Beethoven, Frederic Chopin, Wolfgang Amadeus Mozart and Richard Wagner.

"It is our universal mission and aim to train and make all individuals of global societies realise the management of this planet properly through feeding, treating and providing shelters to the whole population of the planet and make the environment favourable for its inhabitants, so that we as a whole human megastructure could put our collective consciousness and intelligence on the entire exploration of this planet and other universes, thus creating a Universal Neuro-cosmic Civilization."

The main purpose of this book and other volumes of this terrestrial and extraterrestrial "Neurocosmic Brain" is to empower, heal and make the minds of readers and audiences a problem solving and not a problem storing mind. Because social, spiritual and financial problems accumulating in minds are the bigger causes of anxiety, depression poverty and illness. Other than the solution to your personal problems, the

6

volume of this theory will take you to a wonder world of methods, mechanics, of how universe, life and human nature work. While reading this book and other volumes of "Neurocosmic Brain", you will feel like you are on expeditions of exploring life, universe and human nature. After fully exploring all these treasures of real wealth, health, and happiness, you can benefit humanity and yourself in real sense.

In this book, the potential words and ideas based on positive psychology self-help and neuroscience have been used to generate a bioelectrical magnet in your body, soul and mind so that you can attract and leverage goodness, success and achievements through creativity and innovation. By following these rules and methods, you can channel law of attraction in your universal body and mind. The bioelectricity within hidden connotations of words and language used in this theory could also channel natural divine energy flow. You can even gravitate other intelligences around your big mind magnet for the benefit of humanity.

By following the order of divine energy flowing in nature, your bioelectric body could harmonise with this energy system. Influx of oxygen and efflux of carbon dioxide from your lungs and body systems from and into plant leaves via photosynthesis and respiration is one of the biggest examples of this divine energy flowing into our body systems from our ecosystem.

The key components of this neuroscience model include goal setting; the development of our frontal cortex by these executive brain functions make us smarter and civilised. Music therapy, meditation, intuition and brain waves exert a cumulative effect on human epigenetics. As a result, impact of all these factors expresses only the favourable genes conducive to human health, happiness and creativity. Neurocosmic Brain and its innovative publications will help and guide you to achieve universal harmony. Other theories inspiring these books are ocean model of civilisation, according to which, global civilisations could merge through democratic evolution into mega human civilisation for the well-being and general benefit of humanity.

Creative industries network including knowledge-based creative industries could unify the global consciousness and intelligences to fight and head on the common global challenges of pollution, fear of diseases, earthquake, weather, environmental and space catastrophes and to achieve other human rights, and also to combat the fear of terrorism and other undemocratic plights on planet earth.

Mission

Our aim is to enhance the development of the abilities of the global population through the principles of 'Mind Potential Science', and its applications as a philosophy of leadership, self-motivation, individual achievement and societal development.

Our purpose is to enlighten the brains of Global Population, through the fields of Neuropsychology and Success Philosophy. To empower the underprivileged and the people suffering from neurodegenerative diseases, to encourage peoples' knowledge of psychology and mechanics of achieving fitness, wealth, and joy, and to develop an understanding of the purpose of existence of human beings in the Universe.

It is not our intention to dissuade anyone from his/her existing political, religious, economic schools of thought or their professional fields. This book's teachings focus on combatting negative thoughts, desires and impulses and the toxic effects of unnecessary pharmaceutical drugs, etc., from all societies, the effects of which are toxifying the minds and bodies of people and preventing them from appreciating Nature and Life's Potential.

We are committed to promoting awareness of good mental and physical health of individuals in all societies. We do not favour those who waste mental and physical energies through vengefulness, gossip, envy, selfishness and negative competitive behaviour. Instead, we encourage people to be philanthropically creative, focusing thoughts and actions on conquering our nature and fully experiencing the wonders of the Universe.

"Why should we be creative & not competitive?" Neuro-cosmic Idealogy focuses on revolutionising and prospering global societies through creativity and innovation. Neuro-cosmic civilisation will reach its threshold of prosperity when most of the planet's population will start creating art, poetry, music, scientific and technological innovations. According to Neuro-cosmic Ideology, all creative arts and sciences are engines of prosperity.

Creativity is to the ordain randomness of nature and social life in a disciplinary way. Every inventor has to arrange among the chaos of societies. All societies began organising and rearranging themselves according to a set of rules, set up by these inventors. If any society has a good number of inventors in a span of time, it will start to flourish by empowering better organisational structure and will be empowered in every possible way, very smoothly as per the set rules of their inventors.

Professional Fields

We will only invoke creativity and boost one's mental power by teaching them the use of the creative energy present in the Universe to make the mind a powerful 'Mind Magnet'; necessary for harnessing positivity from the Universe in the form of intelligence, healthiness, prosperity, and cheerfulness. You can cultivate this ability; the more it is used, the more you rely on it, and the more it will progress.

Despite the clear benefits, the faculty of creative imagination is one that the majority of people never use. Only a small number of people use it with deliberation and purpose. Those who use this faculty actively and understand its functions are considered 'genius'. By observing and following the rules of mental discipline today, we will emulate the great leaders, scientists, artists, actors, athletes and the originators tomorrow.

Try to imagine the significance and importance of this book's teachings and its potential to increase knowledge and enable achievement in all aspects of life. This knowledge includes the training of individuals associated with educational institutions, from senior to general members of academic staff, who can apply this practical philosophy to themselves, their students, and the wider society, enabling them all to change their lives for a better future.

By following the references and guidance given in this volume you will be able to empower your mind and understand how to develop your 'Mind Magnet' to harness the innovative ideas of your acquired knowledge and use it to develop exquisite abilities ranging from high intelligence levels to the development of skills needed to achieve your wishes of improved health, wealth and happiness.

As authors, we feel that our sheer responsibility is to provide people with proven techniques and tools for personal growth. We have used almost all the methods presented in this book personally— they helped us re-shape our lives and that of others.

To conclude, this book reflects the views and joint opinions of the co-authors.

Chapter 1.

Neuro-Cosmic Ideology Of

Mind Empowerment

"Knowledge has no boundaries; wisdom has no race or nationality."

Our mission, under the umbrella of a 'Global Union of Science and Art Creators', is to universally unify the voices of scientists, artists, poets, musicians and writers to reinforce the power of their written words, sounds, rhythms, melodies and discoveries, etc. to *empower human mind* for the next level of civilisation.

We live in an increasingly challenging world characterised by the rush and race to achieve materialistic goals that have distorted our natural way of thinking and creating — yet, innovations are increasingly valued here. Therefore, meaningful thinking should be used as a vehicle to generating creativity. Hence, we invite scientists, artists, poets, musicians and writers worldwide to join our mission to heal, liberalise, democratise, harmonise and make an ample global population for peace, that is able to conquer the planets and beyond.

Our primary mission should be concentrated on the development of more 'Universal Minds' on this planet in order to enable them to traverse the upcoming global and extra-terrestrial challenges. Our mind is a part-and-parcel of a 'Cosmic Mind'. While the 'Cosmic Mind' in metaphysics is a synonym for 'God's Mind', in the scientific community, it is widely accepted as *'Universal Consciousness'*. Our two universal Neuro-cosmic models of *'Mind Empowerment'* are:

1. Abundance Model
2. Super-consciousness Model

These are both for economic and mental growth. The *'Abundance Model'* is a smart, swift and effective model for mental, social, economic and spiritual growth of individuals and the global communities. The *Super-consciousness Model* on the other hand, is for the development of common minds into transcendental genius minds, encompassing high-dimensional Physics, Philosophy, Metaphysics and Mysticism. This model is for the advancement of human consciousness to the super-consciousness level. It is a process that involves retention of one's awareness not only to operate from the conscious and subconscious levels, but also the super-conscious level. Individuals possessing such a mind, having both abundant and super-consciousness models in their brains, would acquire intelligence of a transcendental genius mind to comprehend and solve the national, global and extra-terrestrial problems.

'Creative *Neuro-Cosmic Industries*', including space research industries, are the foundations of Prof. Anees Akhtar's concept of the *'Neuro-Cosmic Civilisation'*. The structural concepts of these industries should be promoted in global communities. The effects and impact of its outcomes are predicted to be long-lasting on individuals as well as societies. There is a need to introduce the key *Neuro-Cosmic Industries* globally:

1. Writing, painting, art and music industries would propagate knowledge and wisdom to promote, empower, liberalise, harmonise and democratise the minds of global communities.

2. Films, folkdance, Sofiane Kalam and Qawali promote love, harmony and tolerance in societies.

3. Space, Cosmology and Astronomy research and exploration industries have an impact on *'Mind Empowerment'* and on brain neurogenesis of space travellers and explorers.

The founder of *'Neuro-cosmic Civilisation'* *Prof. Anees Akhtar,* appeals to the governments and global communities to implement the ideas of *Neuro-cosmic Industries* in their countries for speedy mental, economic and social growth. For developing countries, a global network of libraries, publishing businesses and trade in art and creative paintings, will promote the Fiction, Non-Fiction and Science Fiction genres of writing and the film industry.

Governments and communities can collaborate to promote trades and business to lay the foundations of the 'Neuro-cosmic Industries' in their countries. This global network of knowledge-promoting business will produce brilliant brains of creative poets, writers, musicians, sculptors, painters, artists and scientists, who will ultimately propagate the message and knowledge of science, art, music to the human brain so dramatically that it will lead to global communities' acquisition of *Mind Empowerment*.

There is a need for an International Global Federation of States to share space research, Space exploration and tourism. In essence, if we are to perceive humanity as a mega-unified structure that includes the developing countries, it would be more beneficial for all nations and governments to be able to cooperate and share their scientists and budgets with all National and International Space Agencies — in order to obtain the benefits of the latest space research for their home countries and the whole world.

1.1 Quantum Approaches of Neuro-cosmic Ideology

According to Prof. Anees Akhtar's Neuro-cosmic ideology, based on metaphysical, quantum and spiritual approaches, the electron is not only a non-living particle, but it is alive inside its quantum field and has a purpose. Due to its certain purpose, it has a definitive direction to go for manifesting the wisdom and intelligence in human life. Within its core, it has an intention and free will and could make choices during its existence.

This approach is implied by 'Neuro-cosmic Ideology' to facilitate the human brain to incorporate chemical signals of musical, spiritual voices and powerful positive words, to get the gene expression on the will of human thoughts and environmental signals, not only at the mercy of predisposed genetic makeup.

According to this theory and model of Mind Empowerment, everything is conscious, which means each particle of matter is conscious, whether it is organic or inorganic. Generally, all humans are conscious of their environment, but not all are much conscious of themselves. If we assume that humans are not conscious of themselves, this may mean that atoms are not conscious of themselves. If we agree to the notion that atoms are conscious, then they must have a sense of 'me'. We also know that for a sense of 'me' to be experienced, atoms require higher organisation of brain and body. If atoms are not fully conscious due to the simplicity of matter, it does not mean that they do not possess intelligence.

We can say intelligence or soul is an invisible part of the space-time continuum. Sometimes the sophisticated minded people and some scientists are generally unaware of intelligence in space-time continuum. Although they have developed their minds to an extraordinary level, they lack spiritual intelligence in a deeper perspective. We can say that they are not fully conscious or transcendental geniuses.

If we can accept this notion that atoms need higher organisation to the level of brain for comprehending consciousness, then we see an extraordinary complexity in the process of our spiritual awakening. It is an extraordinary journey that takes billions and billions of years from an unconscious world of atoms to the awareness of 'oneself'.

We can understand from an evolutionary perspective that intelligence has preceded consciousness, which means consciousness is the building block of 'me'. Today's civilisation of the planet Earth is mentally more developed than the development of consciousness or sense of 'me'. In other words, we can say that our civilisation is lacking spiritual awakening.

We are not spiritually awakened, or we have not yet reached the level of transcendental geniuses, because we focus more on 'Mind Training' rather than awakening our consciousness. After training the minds or raising the intelligence of our students, we ignore the spiritual awakening or sense of 'me' in our students and individuals of the societies. The purpose of spiritual awakening is to recover the healthy balance between intelligence and 'me'. Based on these quantum approaches, for spiritual awakening and consciousness to evolve, we can speculate from a mystical and quantum point of view that, human minds are connected to cosmic or God's mind by sounds and thought waves.

The human mind is a powerful transmission tower, like 1000 TB (Terabytes) memory holding capacity computers. Humans could never build a television or radio transmitting tower, emitting and receiving sounds and thoughts frequencies like the human brain. All these frequencies emitting from human brain are exchanged and proliferated between humans and God's mind.

In another way, we can speculate that according to the quantum and mystical perspective, 'Planet Earth's' total consciousness is strongly connected or bonded with cosmic or God's consciousness.

According to the theories of consciousness presented by most reliable modern Physicists and

Neuroscientists, human brain neurons hold consciousness or memory in their brain as holographic pictures produced by the retina of the human eye and are stored in the human brain by mirror neuron systems. These non-local consciousness or para-psychological messages trigger our brain to produce memory or conscious brain. We can say that our brains are developed by non-local consciousness or mind that is not actually located in the human brain.

These non-local consciousness theories are popular among most of the famous Scientists and Physicists, including Einstein, Nikola Tesla, Michio Kaku, Roger Penrose and other Scientists like David Bohms. All these scientists are looking far beyond to other universal civilisations in different galaxies based on these theories. Today's most popular science fiction films of Hollywood and other industries such as 'Time Travel', 'Mind Gamers' and 'Quantum Dawn', are all based on these concepts of quantum approaches.

Many mystics like Jalaluddin Rumi, Allama Iqbal and Al Ghazali, pointed out the dimension of this spiritual awakening and consciousness located in the human gut brain. You can reach this inner voice of your conscience within your gut by meditation, musical therapies and goal settings discussed in this book, 'Neuroscience of Mind Empowerment and Metacognition'.

Knowledge of Art, music, poetry and literature work together like an enlightened torch to reach this inner voice in the gut brain by meditation and music therapy. By reaching this voice and following its purpose, you can develop a tender heart, genius mind and a great personality in your society.

Chapter 2.

Parapsychology, 'Sixth Sense', Love And Empathy

"Happiness does not rise with standards of living, but only with the standards of loving."

The brain is not hard-wired from birth in the same way as a computer; the brain has the ability to change itself in response to things that happen in our environment. The theory of Epigenetics supports this idea and explains how the environment has profound effects on the expression of genes in their relative environments. Thoughts can change the structure and function of our brain, as well as the expression of genes.

By applying this knowledge and training our brain, we can achieve life's aspirations and help defeat cancer, dementia, eating disorders and other health issues, as well as develop a general sense of wellbeing.

The idea of Neuroplasticity is that our minds are designed to improve as we get older and can be rewired in a useful way that had previously been thought to be impossible – our thoughts and emotions can physically change our brain's chemistry and function. Neuroplasticity can be a kind of 'Superpower' in which success and happiness can be acquired just by reprogramming our brain.

Deepak Chopra writes the following on The Chopra Centre website:

"Regardless of the nature of the genes we inherit from our parents, dynamic change in our thoughts has unlimited influence on our fate."

The following exercises can physically increase our brain strength, size and density:

- ❖ Artificially activate dopamine and endorphins, for creative purposes by applying stimulants of creativity.
- ❖ Consume foods such as blueberries, dark chocolate and green tea.

❖ Taking up yoga, meditation, playing the piano and puzzle games like Sudoku.

2.1 'Sixth Sense' provokes our Creative Imaginative Faculty of Mind

"Imaginations are more important than knowledge."

Creativity is the flash of thoughts in our 'imaginative creative faculty of mind', which are produced in the form of 'hunches' in the conscious mind, utilising brainstorming and mindfulness, for instance, by being alone or sitting in a dark room. The 'sixth sense' creates these flashes in our mind; although scientists have not yet been able to locate them, they can confirm that they definitely have a function in our mind.

To access and use your 'sixth sense', you must activate and train your mind to accept these flashes; you must not ignore them, but utilise and enjoy them and write about them. When they occur, infinite intelligence is activated — our minds are able to purify thoughts and provide solutions to intellectual, business and spiritual issues.

Throughout history, scientists, writers, creators, and thinkers have used their 'sixth sense' effectively and accessed these flashes of thought and inspiration to achieve innovations and patency in research and development – all by using the 'sixth sense' and harnessing the treasures of wisdom and creation from the Universe.

You can follow the different stimulants of creativity; exercising, achieving fame, developing friendship for intellectual purposes, playing games, appreciating food and music and playing a musical instrument – all have the natural ability to produce endorphins and dopamine – the neurotransmitters of wisdom and creativity. The knowledge that you will acquire by engaging in the above and activating the 'creative faculty of your mind', is the most reliable of all forms of knowledge.

The American scientist, Dr Elmer R. Gates, completed 200 patents in which his imagination was stimulated by sitting in a darkened room and waiting for such mental flashes to occur; he earned his living by 'sitting for ideas' for some of America's largest corporations.

2.2 Love and Empathy Flourish in our Brain Regions

Effects of positive thinking, love and empathy reveal in the following areas of the brain:

Limbic Brain

Humans and lower animal species, are born with a limbic brain. It is linked with empathy, love, affection and emotions of nurturing and training their offspring with lifelong skills. Reptiles do not have this specialised brain area and therefore can kill and eat their young and may not always differentiate their young from prey, notwithstanding, for instance, the protective behaviour seen in crocodiles. The presence of the limbic brain in other animals and humans has created empathy and nurturing behaviour towards their upcoming generations.

Vagus Nerves

The two vagus nerves are the longest of the cranial nerves and are sometimes referred to as the 'wandering nerves'. Extending from the brainstem and branching out to multiple organs, including the oesophagus, heart, lungs and digestive system, they form a part of the (involuntary) *autonomic nervous system* that commands unconscious body functions. They also have a role in regulating the immune system.

Charles Darwin called sympathy the strongest of all human instincts. If you are witnessed to suffering or presented with an image of suffering, you will most likely react with compassion; your heart rate will most likely decrease, and you may be impelled to comfort and support the sufferer. If you experience these feelings and physical reactions, it is because humans are 'hard-wired' for it. An empathetic response such as this is activated by the vagus nerves.

Sociopathy

Sociopathy is a psychological condition in which part of the brain responsible for empathetic attitudes is damaged, resulting in a person who cannot maintain normal positive social behaviours. They function on a superficial level, however, appearing and behaving 'normally'.

A similar behavioral condition occurs in sociopathy caused by a brain-damaging incident such as a stroke or accident trauma.

Similarly, when we abuse our power and start ignoring other people's feelings and opinions, we radiate arrogant, ignorant behavior, and it becomes the default nature of our thinking.

Alternatively, empathy, humbleness, and care-giving behaviours provide us with a more authentic and dependable power and trust in society.

Love Follows Spiritual Laws

Love is not a game – you should know the odds. Love is spiritual. Nobody wants fake love — every person wants real love. For real love, you have to learn its spiritual and ethical laws. That is why in human history, spiritual and ethical laws have been the foundation of all great collaborations and romances. When adhering to spiritual and ethical laws, your intuitive heart and neuroplastic brain become expanded, magnified; your relationships are strengthened by spiritual love.

Chapter 3.

How We Feel And Read Other People's Thoughts And Feelings

Charles Darwin – Ideas of thought and feelings

The Universe is made up of thoughts that are combined to make 'infinite intelligence'. According to certain schools of thought, there is a 'Cosmic Mind' formed by the Universe that has the ability to restore, proliferate, perceive and bring forth thoughts to mind according to mental activity. You can switch the frequency of thoughts on and off just by changing what you think and feel; such as creating a feeling of peacefulness and relaxation by listening to soothing music, through meditation, by engaging oneself in creative discussions, or by exercising to feel more invigorated.

According to a Japanese Scientist, Dr Masaru Emoto, "Words have power in themselves." His research suggested that molecules of water are affected by our thoughts, words and feelings. As water makes up to 70% of our body, bad words negatively affect the structure of water, whereas good words help – as in Dr Emoto's snowflake crystals, by taking shape of beautiful patterns when exposed to words of love and gratitude —by inference creating beautiful water molecules.

According to Dr Emoto, words are an expression of the soul and the condition of our soul has a large impact on water. The language we use and the words we choose are vitally important. Verbal abuse can have dangerous and damaging psychological effects – "words and language have tremendous power, as does the intent behind them."

The tone of the voice also has the ability to heal. Certain voices can keep your attention, whereas others don't. When we listen to a wonderful rich resonant voice, it can feel very therapeutic. If someone says something loving and kind to you in a gentle tone of voice, it is likely to make you feel good. But if someone yells at you in a harsh way, it tends to have a destructive effect.

The words we say originate from our thoughts. Thoughts can be toxic or good, depending on the way you behave and how you think and feel; so, try to avoid toxic thoughts — they are more harmful effect than an unhealthy diet. Our hijacked amygdala is not always prone to sustain good thoughts because in the history of evolution, negative emotions, like fear and anger, have great *survival* value, which impels a threatened animal to fight.

According to Charles Darwin, our ability to send and read emotions has played an enormous role in human evolution, both in creating and maintaining social order, particularly with negative feelings; we usually respond more strongly to someone who is angry than to someone who is in a good mood, creating a loop of negativity or rage.

How did we become Spiritual Survival Machines on this Planet?

Our chemical and electromagnetic nature has made us a spiritual survival machine on this Planet, and a sub-total of the subatomic manifestation of the bi-symmetrical nature of the Universe. Our brain is a powerful 'receiving and transmitting tower'; our feet and toes, hands and fingers, are like sensors that detect signals from the Earth and Universe, passing them via the nervous system to the brain, broadcasting feelings and thoughts through the brain that are detected from the environment. The two symmetries of the bi-symmetrical Universe is analogous with the way the brain's left and right hemispheres are joined by the white & grey matter; by chemical bonding, the junction between the two hemispheres connects the two halves of the brain by the neural connections. We have 86 billion neurons in both halves of the brain. Each neuron can connect with other neurons; there are from 5,000 to 10,000 different connections. The number of neurons in the human brain is more than all the stars of the Universe. The neuron is the basic information-processing unit that is responsible for understanding, memories and our behaviour. Interconnected neurons make up the structure of the brain. As the signals pass on, the neurons create a network by firing and wiring between these neurons, creating our personalities and helping us to perceive the world around us.

When we try to remember the name of a person or recall what we read in a book, a neural network will develop a memory of this through neurotransmitters that build the chemical and electrical signals to bridge the gap between two neurons.

3.1 Nature of the Human Brain

❖ Is the most complex and mysterious machine in the Universe?

❖ Its power is many-fold higher than a basic modern computer.

❖ Its storage capacity is about 1,000 terabytes.

❖ It does millions of different things at once.

❖ It stores the day's events at night and can catalogue, archive and recall memories at a later date.

❖ You cannot hear, feel or think about it – the brain mostly acts subconsciously; but the more you actively exercise your brain, the more it will benefit you.

❖ It is the organ that controls and operates the neural systems of the human body, which is made up of around 80 billion to 100 billion nerve cells (neurons).

The brain is used to:

❖ Store memories.

❖ Control our body's functions.

❖ Communicate and react to our surroundings.

❖ Give us the power to think.

Neurochemistry:

The Human brain has the following compositions:

❖ 78% water

❖ 10% lipids

❖ 8% proteins

❖ 1% carbohydrate

❖ 2% solid organics

❖ 1% inorganic salts

Amygdala:

Socially active people have the largest amygdala; the part of the brain that plays a big role in social and mental wellbeing – therefore it is important to build more grey matter in the brain by understanding more about the world around us.

Earth's first life forms were prokaryotes. Several billion years later, human beings have evolved to become complex multi-cellular forms. We evolved into advanced homo-sapien forms by developing, adapting and controlling our minds and bodies. Two hundred thousand years ago when humans learned to command fire, they started cooking the meat of hunted animals that led to less energy required for digestion. Consequently, this led to increased blood supply to the brain instead of the stomach. This excess blood in our brain has allowed it to adapt and to grow in size and functionality, therefore increasing the speed and nature of our thoughts. It is by this evolution that the human race became the dominant species on this planet.

Over the past few centuries, our intelligence has sharpened with the advancement of technology and medicine. The brain is split into two parts:

* Left Hemisphere.
* Right Hemisphere.

Left side of the brain controls:

* Speech
* Writing
* Logics

Right side of the brain controls:

* Creativity
* Emotions
* Information

Information is processed as quickly as 120 meters/second, or 268 miles per hour, in the brain. The weight of the human brain is about 1.4 kg. It is relatively bigger than that of almost any other animal. As mentioned, the human mind is the most powerful 'receiving and transmitting tower' in the Universe. Around 60,000 thoughts are perceived and proliferated by it per day — by knowing our feelings we can control our thoughts.

Humans are curious about the world around them. They not only accumulate extra food, like lower animals, but they want to know what lies over the horizon to attain the pure joy of it. Even though not all humans may be great thinkers, they can understand the concepts of truth, justice or honesty.

Creativity is a fundamental part of our nature and human beings are in constant search for new ways to do things and for new things to do.

Societies devoting a huge amount of energy on science, art and literature advance further than those that ignore these endeavours – as creativity breeds more creativity. We should adopt the habit of creative thinking.

Chapter 4.

Chemical/Electromagnetic Nature Of The Human Mind And Body

Newton's law of attraction and prevailing love in nature and the Universe.

All chemical and electromagnetic processes of the human body and brain function are similar to all electrical and magnetic entities and bodies in the Universe; from atom to Solar System, milkyways galaxies and all life on this Planet – they are all linked to each other through chemical and electromagnetic attraction and communication.

Similarly, as in the human body, plants and animal's 'cell signalling mechanisms', and chemical communication between microbes in the form of 'Quorum Sensing', are the greatest manifestation of the law of attraction and love in Nature and the Universe; the same law co-ordinates the galaxies, Solar Systems, and life on our beautiful Planet. This is the law of attraction

44

or love in nature or Newton's 2nd Law of Gravity.

4.1 Scattered Matter in the Universe

After the 'Big Bang', matter has been scattered throughout the Universe and is present in living and non-living things to the point that it is difficult to fully understand its mechanism of action on living and non-living things. In some situations, it is partially explained and understood at its atomic and molecular level. However, still a lot of work has to be done in Physics, Chemistry and Biology to understand its mysterious mechanism of action completely.

New branches of these sciences, like genetic engineering and nanotechnologies, will use much of its theoretical and practical approaches to make innovations in the coming decades – which will open up some new debates among researchers – to enable us to understand the mechanisms of action in living and non-living things.

Still, the issues of protein-folding and the

mechanisms of division of the AIDS' virus proteins – and artificial and therapeutic repairs of damaged DNA – may remain a mystery for the foreseeable future.

We have not yet harnessed the full form of chemical energy, as produced in the chemical forms in plants, insects, microbes and animal and human tissues, in the form of alkaloids, steroids, proteins, hormones, antibodies and antibiotics.

Should we be able to harness all chemical forms of energy from the above sources in the future, we would be able to find the cure for Cancer, AIDS, Hepatitis, Arthritis and various cardiovascular diseases as well as for many genetic disorders to which certain people are predisposed.

4.2 Quantum Physics and Consciousness

Human consciousness has not yet fully understood the dynamic functions of the different energy forms in the Universe, which is in the form of energy beams of 'infinite intelligence'. This energy may be in the form of photons, quarks, waves, chemical or electromagnetic forms. This energy sometimes combines chemically and electromagnetically to form proteins, hormones, antibodies, antibiotics and vaccines.

When human consciousness fully understands the different forms of energy and can harness their dynamic uses, the human mind, culture, societies and health conditions will advance greatly by adopting new technologies, new ways of thinking and beliefs in science, art, culture and philosophy. When 'infinite intelligence' and human consciousness become harmonised, it harnesses its form and enables the creation of novel innovations. Many inventions and creations come into existence when we are intensely focused on thoughts, utilising the 'sixth sense' to boost our creative imaginative faculty. We are medically, technologically and culturally conscious or hyperconscious, in as much as we know about the different energy forms responsible for dynamically activating in the Universe. Harnessing this energy, either in atomic, molecular or chemical form, gives us consciousness and improves humans medically, technologically and culturally, enabling us to empower our minds and experience a new consciousness of thought, hidden in the folded energy beams in the Universe.

Chapter 5.

Knowledge Enhances Our Emotional Intelligence And Outlook

Emotional intelligence and the value of acquiring and promoting knowledge.

"Dig deeper into the emotional reservoir."

Psychologists have proven that people who had *actively* tried to improve their personalities got more jobs as executives than those who had inferior personalities but greater abilities – it is said that in China, 'a man who cannot smile must not open the shop'.

A smile is magnetic, and a frown is un-magnetic (not attractive); it takes more facial muscles to frown than it does to smile.

5.1 Optimistic vs Pessimistic

People who are optimistic, bright and hopeful are

more popular and appealing to others – people want to be around them. Pessimists constantly bemoan their losses in life; always dwelling on the bad things that have happened to them or that they expect to happen. Be optimistic rather than pessimistic and avoid talking about sickness, accidents, failure and unhappiness – instead talk about pleasure and happy events.

Reasons to be an optimist:

* Optimists live longer than pessimists and have a 50% lower risk of dying early than pessimists.
* Optimists have fewer physical and emotional or health problems. They suffer less pain and they have increased energy and generally feel more peaceful, happier and calmer than pessimists. Being an optimist protects you from illness.

A positive attitude is so important because it boosts our immune systems, thus enabling us to fight illness. Positive people were found to be more resistant to the influenza virus than negative people when exposed to an infectious environment. Research studies into positive attitudes have revealed positivity to be the best prevention against heart diseases.

According to Dr David Hamilton, people who are most satisfied with their lives live longer because satisfaction in life means taking interest in life and the means of happiness.

5.2 Complaining is a Contagious Behaviour

Complaining about things and people affects those around us. When we complain around people, we trigger their dominant complaining instinct. They are also likely to find fault with life and the world in general. It is therefore a contagious behaviour that affects the people around us.

Our keen observations and research show that when we have a certain goal and imagine our destiny, our minds focus on that goal and achieving targets associated with that of the destiny. However, as soon as we get bored and lose sight of our destiny, we suddenly view life more negatively and start complaining about trivial matters, opposing things and starting petty arguments.

One thing that can boost your morale is to share your power, wealth, happiness and status with other people. It's possible to achieve more happiness by giving away money to people and charities; by showing this generosity (even if it's a small amount of your salary) you share your strength, knowledge, happiness and other attributes and experience a boost in your morale and feelings of contentment.

Similarly, our positive attitude towards our aging mind and body reduces the incidence of high blood pressure (hypertension) and heart diseases. By visualising the happier moments of our younger life, we can reduce the physiological and anatomical aging process, which will enable us to feel sharper, look younger and feel more energised. The sense of gratitude and visualising the positive effects of achieving a goal can help at boosting your potential to do more and achieve more; be courteous and kind when dealing with others, and eventually, you will reap the benefits of doing so.

5.3 Interior vs Exterior of your Personality

Your exterior personality is that which you show the world. It is important, this profile should present a true and honest, well-groomed being with a cheerful, happy countenance; displaying the qualities of a 'million-dollar personality'.

If the interior side is coloured by thoughts of unhappiness, fear, failure, worry, hate, envy, and revenge. Reservations will soon reflect this negative mental attitude to the outer world, and it will drive people away from you.

"What you habitually think, you will become."

The interior aspects of ourselves have had long-lasting effects on our personality – therefore, dig deeper into the emotional reservoir and keep your thoughts beautiful and inspiring, and your exterior personality will also evolve to be beautiful.

Build positive qualities like friendliness, trust, confidence, loyalty, cheerfulness, happiness, honesty, goodness, trustfulness and clarity in your mind and they will shine through and be obvious for all to see. There is present a natural system of accountability, judgement, punishment or reward in your Parasympathetic Nervous System:

"God will forgive your sins, but your nervous system won't."

5.4 Value of Acquiring and Promoting Knowledge

The ability to learn, pass on knowledge, and teach it to others allows knowledge to be disseminated. Thus, a civilisation can be created.

Civilisation distinguishes the human species from all other forms of life. Every society needs to encourage and promote learning amongst its citizens or risk being left behind and eventually dominated by neighbouring societies. There is more awareness and consciousness in families, societies and states where reading and study are common.

5.5 Speed-Reading Promotes Retention of Knowledge

The American educator Evelyn Wood, developed the basic techniques of speed-reading in the 1950's. She set up institutes for students to develop the ability to read hundreds of words per minute — many business people and politicians have studied her methods. American Presidents, Jimmy Carter and John F. Kennedy are regarded as famous speed-readers.

5.6 Quantum Words and Knowledge Energy

The words of all knowledge preserved in books, arts and technology are quantum in nature, and their energy is widespread in human intelligence. It is also widespread in the universe in the form of particles of infinite intelligence. These quantum words of knowledge are perceived into human intelligence through five senses. After proliferating into the brain and the heart, this energy of words purifies the circulating blood in the body. It also purifies and energises the body organs and muscles by their big energy fields affecting each body cell. The intelligence is produced by words that function as quantum particles of energy in the cells of our body.

We know that the human mind and body structures are built like a complex machine. This machine needs solid food and water for digestion, absorption, circulation and excretion. This body also needs spiritual and quantum energy of words and knowledge to harmonise and logicalise with the environment and society. This energy of words and knowledge also helps maintain our inner homeostasis, metabolism and intrinsic chemical reactions. The energy helps maintain a balance between inside and outside of our complex human machine. In human civilisation, this knowledge energy of quantum words has been preserved in the form of books, art, technology, music, paintings, sculptures and also in the form of spiritual and ethical knowledge.

When the human mind reads or perceives a word or a voice from a great book or coherent speech, these words, due to their electrical and quantum nature, produce turbulence or self-talk. This self-talk produces logic within the mind and the heart. This makes this machine logical and harmonious with its internal and external environment. After proliferation into the brain and the heart, this energy merges into the blood chemistry of this human machine.

This spiritual cleaning of human machine makes us wise and honest and compatible to the societies and environments, and as a whole with the great universal structure. If any of us is holding confusion or impurities in our thoughts and heart, we ought to dig deeper into the science, art, musical and spiritual knowledge to get rid of all the confusion and impurities from our mind, heart and soul to empower our inner and outer balance, which is very important for human dignity, purity and personal growth. This is the only way to personal growth and universal exploration.

This will bring peace, prosperity, curiosity and creativity in our societies. It is our social and moral duty to promote good educational and research institutions, widespread global system of digital and physical libraries to build great human civilisation. We should promote and build great scientific and literary platforms for our youngsters where they can practice and perform their unique literacy, scientific and creative talent to manifest themselves in this challenging world.

Chapter 6.

Achieve Your Goal And

Reach Your Destiny

"Don't just make a living, make a life."

Our Lecture Series Output

When we came to believe in ourselves, we started writing and speaking to tell others about our feelings and experiences. Other people around us gained inspiration from our ideas, growing wisdom and concepts. They started to believe our view that we can use this knowledge and wisdom to strengthen faith in ourselves, other people and *'Infinite Intelligence'*.

Our minds are capable of influencing our fate and wellbeing. Our audience started to apply the principles we taught them, and they found that these belief systems and faith in their subconscious mind could combat diseases and attain goals in their lives.

These elaborated techniques of visualisation, affirmation and autosuggestion strengthen people's 'faith', and help them build a strong fabric of mind for positive thinking, enhancing their mind, body and the world around them. This subsequently leads to demand for more explanation of the truth about the nature of the human mind and elicits more and more from the *universal infinite intelligence*' in the form of health, wealth, prosperity, happiness and strong relationships.

Most of the people to whom we have been presenting these concepts started believing that these are real principles. Consequently, by applying these principles, they started utilising the maximum capacity of their minds, which for a normal person is usually not more than 5-10%, in their whole life.

These principles of mind empowerment science, epigenetics, neuroplasticity, mindfulness, and music therapy have the potential of maximising one's mental capability and capacity, to take control of your whole body's complex systems in a more harmonious manner.

We can control our mind, which is the monitor of our body-systems, i.e. digestive, respiratory, circulatory, nervous and endocrine systems. Consequently, our body systems are more harmonious and healthier, extending longevity by cultivating a positive mental attitude. You can combat illness and pain by an optimistic approach towards the environment by expanding your positive 'Mind Magnet' or Neuroplastic Nature of your mind.

By positive attitude and by the habit of gratitude, you can detoxify any relationship around you, can synchronise any heart and get the benefit of new constructive reactions due to the pleasurable feeling of the inner balance.

Part Two of Lecture

The second principle and rule that we applied on ourselves and taught others to get the maximum achievement is to utilise your subconscious mind; write down affirmations daily and follow them and write down the short-term and long-term goals to be achieved in your path to a big destiny. The most important and having the highest impact on Man's health, wealth, happiness and abundance, are the influences of brainstorming, meditation and visualisation, which set up your destiny or major goals in your life that will move your mind towards your objective, without any fear or hesitation. If you have a properly written goal and destiny that you want to reach over a period of 1-3 years you will have a strong & positive impact on your body's immune system and your willpower. This action will reduce all negative emotions like fear and procrastination from the mind; your predominant thoughts will be goal-oriented and will alter your whole mental and genetic makeup.

You will start making new perceptions of the world around you. Then you will become the successful *'captain and commander'* of your life and fate. You will soon feel that you have designed a ladder to climb to the 'beautiful palace' of your goals. Your subconscious mind and universal infinite intelligence and cosmic mind or paranormal divine energy, has started autopilot work to achieve successes in your life. This is how the Universe is leveraged — the law of attraction starts working — and God, the 'universal infinite intelligence', starts bestowing the blessings of wisdom, health, wealth, prosperity and abundance on such a mind.

In addition, you will feel a 'Heaven on Earth' by achieving this inner balance in the heart and mind. This is the way of the wise, noble, honest and 'Million-Dollar Minds'. You may have everything from prosperity, affluence and abundance in life, but also have the blessings of bliss and tranquillity.

Consequently, you will have successfully shifted yourself from a material survival machine to a spiritual being with a higher purpose in life.

Purposeful Life

The third principle to apply to yourselves is to set up a mission in your life because mission-orientated people are more resilient to adverse conditions. They work hard to reach their goal and complete their mission that strengthens their immune system and extends their longevity of life.

By setting up these noble goals, you set up a chain of constructive chemical reactions in your mind and body, and your subconscious will start surveillance of the conscious mind to fulfil these goals.

Only the mission-orientated life can teach you the higher purpose of human beings in the Universe. This is the secret of finding the truth lying over the horizon of universal mysteries, which should be explored by the human mind. Hence, you set up a written goal and destiny to reach; and you live a purposeful life, and you automatically develop the habits of success and million-dollar-mindedness in yourself.

Your mission in life may be philanthropy, of serving humanity with the ideas of loving, peace, prosperity, abundance, affluence, tranquillity and bliss in every human life, or something else. However, if you have no such written and instructed navigator in your mind, you will have to wander, and chances are you will be deviated from the goal and destiny, and you will be unsuccessful and lost in your life.

Chapter 7.

Epigenetics: How Your Thoughts Can Alter Your Genetic Makeup

The New Science of Self-Empowerment:
Epigenetics is a new revolutionary field in Biology. Epigenetics means control above genetics. It means that environmental influences, like nutrition, stress and emotions can modify genes without changing their basic blueprint. These modifications of genes can be passed on to future generations, as the DNA blueprints are passed on via the double helix.

When DNA is uncovered, the cell makes the copy of the exposed gene, which means that the activity of the gene is controlled by the presence or absence of the covering proteins, which are controlled by environmental signals.

Epigenetic research predicts how environmental signals control the activity of genes. According to this research, the information goes to regulatory protein, to DNA, to RNA, resulting in protein synthesis. Epigenetic research has shown us that there are two mechanisms by which organisms pass on hereditary information. These mechanisms provide a way for scientists to study both the contributions of genes and control of epigenetics in human behaviour. If we only focus on DNA blueprints, then the influence of environment becomes impossible to understand.

Research shows that information that controls biology starts with environmental signals that in turn control the activity of regulatory proteins of DNA. Regulatory protein directs the activity of genes. DNA, RNA and protein functions are the same as described in the DNA model. As the flow of information is no longer unidirectional, RNA could go against the predicted flow of information and can rewrite the DNA programme. This is called *reverse transcriptase*, which is used by the AIDS virus to command the infected DNA cells.

It is known that epigenetic changes in the DNA molecule, such as adding or removing methyl chemical groups, can influence the binding of regulatory proteins. Proteins are also responsible for the predicted flow of information, as protein antibodies in immune cells are involved with changing the DNA in the cells that synthesise them.

As environmental signals affect us epigenetically, regulatory proteins can 'dial up' and create 2,000 or more variations of protein from the same blueprint. Modification in genes by environmental signalling can pass from one generation to the next generation.

Bruce Lipton performed an experiment on mice that was predisposed to cardiovascular disease, diabetes and cancer. The mice were fed with a methyl group-rich supplement. Since methylation of DNA can silence or modify gene activity and is involved with epigenetic modifications, when methyl groups attach to gene DNA, it changes the way the regulatory chromosomal protein binds to the DNA molecule. When protein binds tightly to the gene, it can be removed by the environmental signals, so the gene can be read. This is why methylation of DNA can inactivate or modify gene activity; this chemical application subsequently prevented the mice from developing the cancers.

The optimistic and pessimistic attitude 'taught' in childhood, and 'learned' in stressful environmental circumstances, also affects telomerase activity. If we stay optimistic, it extends telomere length, which enhances health and extends life.

Extending the length of telomeres by the activity of enzymes, called telomerase, could increase the vitality and productivity of stem cells. Enhanced telomerase activity is the 'Fountain of Youth' and promotes a long and healthy life. Different life experiences or events happening in life can stimulate or suppress telomerase activity. Stressful parental development, child abuse, domestic violence, post-traumatic stress disorder, nutritional deficiencies and lack of love all inhibit telomerase activity.

On the other hand, exercise, good nutrition, a positive outlook in life, living in happiness and gratitude, experiencing love and affection; all these factors enhance telomerase activity and promote a long and healthy life.

In a recent study, it was found that breast cancer patients who were involved in mindfulness meditation tended to preserve telomere length, whilst in a telomere control group, those without these interventions resulted in shorter telomere length; research on the telomere shows that 2% of the genome that encodes protein has a big impact on health and disease.

In an experiment done on cultured cells, it was found that approximately 50 generations of cells are produced before their telomeres are lost. DNA replication then produces defective protein, which causes the cell's death and compromises its ability to divide further.

Humans have a finite life span, determined by how many times the stem cells divide and replace billions of cells that die every day.

Elaine Fox, in her book 'Sunny Brain and Rainy Brain', explains that there is a strong relationship between our genetic makeup and the environment we live in. It means that the switching on or switching off, or down-regulation or up-regulation of our genes are dependent on the environmental signals that they 'dial up' or switch up.

In other words, our genes do not operate in isolation, but start signalling when interacting with the environment, so genes and the environment *can* work interdependently to develop our personality and outlook. The technologies of modern molecular genetics, neuroscience, and psychology have been much synergised to understand this mechanism. Consequently, if we develop a tendency to re-train our brains, we can alter our genetic code by transmitting positive thoughts.

The following are the main examples and evidences of expression of genes dependent on the kind of environment. Genes are a specific sequence of DNA. Information in DNA is stored in the form of DNA codes; these codes are made up of four chemical bases which are called nucleotides; linked together as:

A=T (Adenine=Thymine)

G≡C (Guanine≡Cytosine)

When one base joins ribose sugar and one phosphate molecule, they are called nucleotides. These four nucleotides given above are core structures of DNA. The gene is the particular sequence of these nucleotide pairs. As DNA inherits from generation after generation, the sequence of DNA remains constant. When genes have variations in their structure, they produce abnormal effects (mutations) in the body and brain. Gene mutations can have positive or negative effects.

These variations in genes are known as Single Nucleotide Polymorphism (SNP). These variations can develop into a disease or any specific personality trait. For example, the serotonin transporter gene and dopamine receptor gene affect the serotonin and dopamine level in the brain.

These two SNP changes in genes affect the mental states of the patient. The way by which these particular neurotransmitter systems affect the specific gene is known as the *candidate gene approach*. The person carrying vulnerability genes has a particular SNP gene.

People carrying a vulnerability gene of lung cancer have a higher risk of developing lung cancer when they are exposed to carcinogenic compounds that are consumed in food or through smoking.

Similarly, a vulnerability gene of anxiety will develop anxiety when susceptible people are exposed to stress and trauma.

COMT gene (catechol-O-methyltransferase):

A research study performed on the COMT gene by Danny Weinberger shows that the COMT gene is involved in the production of dopamine balance in the brain where dopamine maintains the pleasure system. Too much dopamine can cause schizophrenia.

Research studies show that insufficient COMT gene has poor activity in the brain's pre-frontal cortex, so variation in the COMT gene can be the cause of schizophrenia.

MAOA gene (Monoamine Oxidase A):

In another scientific study on the effect of the gene and environment on personality traits, it was shown that:

Abused children with the low expression of MAOA gene develop serious mental health problems and become involved in criminal and antisocial behaviour. On the other hand, children having the high expression of MAOA gene did not develop any serious mental health problems, even though they had experienced serious abuse.

Epigenetic modifications are stable and they are passed to future generations. They are changed in response to environmental stimuli. Epigenetics has influenced all aspects of Biology and has developed into one of the most important fields in biological science.

David Hamilton (2009) explained that genes can

be activated by the state of mind. If you have a happier and positive state of mind, new genes will start signalling, and new beneficial proteins will be produced for your mind and body.

But if you have pessimistic and toxic thoughts, the genes will signal the toxic proteins to the brain and body. Hence by changing our mind, we can change our body at the subatomic and cellular level. As when a gene is switched on, a new protein is produced — this protein may be involved in the construction of new cells and tissues, new bone cells, blood cells or may be used to form immune systems.

This protein produced by the activation of genes can be an enzyme that can catalyse other chemical reactions in formulations of new proteins and molecules. For example — pepsin, an enzyme produced in the stomach, can convert food into digestive substances.

This protein produced by gene activation may be hormones, whose function is signalling to other cells. Activation of genes by signals of our mind can produce hormones, such as growth hormones that help in healing wounds and other damaged tissues. It is found that mental and emotional stress reduces the level of growth hormone at wound sites.

It is found that due to stress, over one hundred genes are *down-regulated.* Similarly, over 70 genes are *upregulated* by cultivating pleasure and optimism and by maintaining a grateful attitude. Therefore, when over 70 genes are down-regulated, it diminishes the healing of wounds by lack of growth hormones.

Consequently, cultivating a feel-good and optimistic attitude increases the up-regulation of growth hormones at wound sites, as our thoughts affect our genes that are signalling for proteins. Mixtures of genes are involved in different functions.

If we have a family history of an oncogene (cancer-causing) or a cardiac failure gene and if we keep worrying about their presence in our makeup, the risk is likely that we *will be* the victim of cancer or heart disease.

But even if we have those oncogenes in our genetic makeup but never concern ourselves about them and keep ourselves in good dietary, environmental and positive psychological conditions, then there are few chances of activation of these genes, and we would be safe from this genetic risk; our 'instruction' can turn down the bad genes. Like it is said, "Sometimes ignorance is a blessing."

On the other hand, our thoughts also influence the growth of stem cells because stem cells have DNA that is controlled by environmental signals. When the genes are activated, stem cells can become bone cells, immune cells, skin cells, heart cells, blood cells, or neurons – stress, though, can interfere with neurogenesis.

Embryonic stem cells can be transplanted into the liver or heart, which can re-grow the damaged part of the organs. When a skin wound heals, stem cells travel *from* bone marrow into skin cells.

Stem cells can also travel *to* bone marrow and into the heart cells to regenerate damaged heart muscle.

Chapter 8.

Neuroplasticity: Rewire And Alter The Structure Of Your Brain

"The brain is not 'hard-wired'."

According to Norman Doidge in his book, 'The Brain that Changes itself', Neuro means neurons or nerve cells in our brain or nervous system. Plastic means changeable, malleable, or modifiable. Neuroplasticity then means that 'we see with our brain, not with our eyes'. Neuroplasticity has implications for our understanding of how relationships, love, sex, greed, addiction, culture, technology, learning and psychotherapies change our brain.

Neuroplasticity is the power of the mind that is capable of changing, expanding and constantly enhancing, with a positive interaction with the environment. Even a brain that has sustained injuries can rebuild itself by positive affirmations and by thinking about a certain goal and can rewire the whole brain.

Now we know that we are not at the mercy of the genetically predetermined brain makeup; we can alter our brain structure and function by our positive and optimistic thinking.

Research studies proved by brain scanning that many OCD patients, stroke victims and musicians have changed their brain for the better by applying the principles of *self-directed* neuroplasticity. Previously, it was thought that the brain was fixed and hard-wired and that the teen years and mid-'20s were the final stages of the brain's development.

Now, new research in the field of neuroscience shows that the brain is malleable and is plastic in nature. If it could be rewired according to our behaviour towards our environment and instincts, it means we can make new adaptive changes in our brain by adjusting ourselves in better environments and social situations. By learning new skills, we make new connections in our memories, and we keep it changing throughout our life by learning new skills, languages and new ways of doing things. By learning new skills, we make new memory connections in our minds and continue this process throughout our whole life by learning innovative skills, language proficiency and by practising new methodologies.

On the other hand, foods such as blueberries, green tea, dark chocolate, vegetables, fish, fruits and nuts, enhance the building up of new neuro-connections in the brain, making it flourish.

In some neurodegenerative diseases and brain-damage injuries, the brain is able to respond to music therapies, brain wave entrainment therapies, meditation and by mindfulness practises. By setting up achievable goals and aims in our lives, we could boost the plasticity of the brain and completely change its structure and functioning.

In a comparative research study reported by Elaine Fox in her book 'Sunny Brain and Rainy Brain', London's black cab taxi drivers' fMRI scans showed that the back part of their brain, the hippocampus was larger than that of the general population. This part of the brain is associated with navigation in birds, animals and humans. Taxi drivers have to learn over 25,000 different London streets to pass their taxi-driving test (The Knowledge). That is why the size of their hippocampus grows bigger with more time spent in the taxi profession.

8.1 Professional Musicians and Brain Neuroplasticity

Studies utilising high-resolution MRI brain scans of professional musicians show that the brains of musicians and non-musicians differ in significant ways. Music performance is regarded as one of the most impressive of all human achievements.

Studies on MRI-scanned brains of musicians and non-musicians show that the brain areas involved in hearing complex sounds are much larger in musicians than those of the non-musicians. Research shows that music practice increases their relevant brain regions.

With the discovery of neuroplasticity, we can now understand that the brain is capable of more flexibility. We have rejected the old notion that the brain is fixed and hard-wired. We know now that our brain never ceases to respond to new skills and our environmental stimulus; it is learning from birth and continues until we die. Neuroscience research shows that a complex network of neurons and pathways of nerve fibres inside our head are constantly responding, adapting and rearranging themselves. This flexibility presents us with great opportunities to change our outlook.

The brain's plasticity increases when we challenge our brain with new things, beliefs and ways of doing things differently. If we do not use parts of our brain, these brain areas will gradually be taken over by other functions. Still, if we make efforts, even deeply embedded circuits have the potential to change.

As in the past, there have been evidences for neuroplasticity, so this science will make it possible in the future for new treatments for the range of degenerative brain disorders like

Parkinson's, Alzheimer's and other neurological conditions. It is speculated that this power may also cure mental health problems such as anxiety and depression of neuroplasticity.

Dr David Hamilton, in 'How your Mind Can Heal Your Body?', reported several different successful experiments on different groups of patients and the population generally. He found that our five senses and 'sixth sense' perception and conceiving stimulus in our mind increases our brain plasticity. When we perceive a new idea in our mind and start nurturing it, it causes millions of neurons or brain cells to fire and wire together, which enhances the capacity of our mind to enhance.

Meditation increases the thickness of the pre-frontal cortex in the brain. Visualising good health, wealth, wellness, happiness, prosperity, and wisdom alters our brain's microscopic structure and starts signalling new genes for beneficial proteins. We can thus experience changes in our genetic makeup at the subatomic level.

These new neuro connections start dissolving stress, trauma and start regenerating the damaged part of the brain that is injured. This is called the neurogenesis or rewiring of our brain by positive thinking. By surrendering our ego and prestige, replacing the emotions of hate, envy, judgement and competitive emotions with creative constructive criticism and curiosity by maintaining our joint struggle to conquer the mysteries of the Universe, our brain plasticity will expand. Neuroscience research shows that our brain has the capacity of neurogenesis to all areas of our brain.

As mentioned earlier, some antioxidant foods like blueberries, dark chocolate, green tea, and other nutrients available at herbal and synthetic drug stores can help to boost mental capacity and plasticity. The following amino acid supplements have powerful effects on repairing the brain atrophy caused by stress and have amazing effects to enhance brain plasticity:

❖ **Ginkgo Biloba:** Increases brain oxygen uptake. Helps neural growth.

- ❖ **L. Arginine:** Lowers blood pressure. Assists with increasing low libido.
- ❖ **Glycine:** Helps optimise sugar levels and sleep.
- ❖ **Acetylcholine (ACh):** A neuromodulator that can help repair brain atrophy and control motivation, arousal and attention.
- ❖ **DL - phenylalanine:** Helps treat chronic pain depression, attention deficit-hyperactivity disorder (ADHD), Parkinson's disease, alcohol withdrawal symptoms and a skin disease called vitiligo.
- ❖ **GABA:** Improves mood, relieves anxiety, improves sleep and treats ADHD.
- ❖ **L-glutathione:** Treating alcoholism, weakened immune systems, memory loss, Alzheimer's and Parkinson's diseases.
- ❖ **Ginseng:** Helps in cognitive functioning.

8.2 Power of Your Faith can Cure and Dissolve Illness

David Hamilton explained that the power of faith has a placebo effect in dissolving illness. If we have strong faith and believe that our subconscious mind has all capabilities to bring out all the solutions to our spiritual and professional problems, then we can also apply this power of belief and faith in curing illnesses. For example, if we believe in certain drugs that they will cure our illnesses even though that drug has no chemical substances to cure that disease, our faith in drugs will make our mind produce that active chemical in our brain that will actually eradicate that kind of illness.

It has been proven by testing on some patients that are merely strengthening their belief and faith in drugs to cure illness will produce healing compounds from the brain that could bring the remedy, even if the patients are given placebo drugs. Our mind itself is a big 'pharmacy' of many healing compounds/drugs that even pharmaceutical companies have not yet made. Such drugs that a mind may produce just by strengthening faith on the remedy for illness means that the brain governs the placebo effects of the drugs.

The brain itself can produce any compound, from

painkillers to antidepressants; even spiritual healing methods have strong placebo effects on our mind and body.

8.3 Visualisation and Affirmation

In his book 'How your mind can heal your body?', David Hamilton describes much experimental evidence of the effects of visualisation and affirmation that help boost the plasticity of mind and healing.

If you focus on a specific part of the body that is connected to the brain, as nerves connect the brain, to the skin, muscles, bones, tendons and internal organs – for example, if we imagine moving our fingers, toes or tongue – the area of the brain that governs these parts of the body is activated. As the nerves connect the brain to the muscles, the muscles also get stronger when we merely *imagine* using them.

Scientists tested the volunteers for different experiments, and they found that individuals who were doing real exercise of different parts of the body, contrasted with those who were only imagining that exercise. It was found that those who were just doing the imaginary exercise developed strength in those parts of the body.

The athletic community has long known that muscles can be affected by brain visualisation strategies. Research has proven that the brain is stimulated by visualisation, which in turn stimulates optimal muscle performance. If an athlete regularly visualises running for a world record at the required speed, it is likely that muscles will develop and perform differently compared to those who did not use visualising techniques. It is found that just watching someone exercise can affect our brain and muscles.

A research experiment was performed on volunteers who were only allowed to watch people moving their hands, mouth and feet. By scanning the volunteer's brains, it was found that areas that control hands, mouth and feet movements appeared to be activated and subsequently became more developed. If we watch an image while performing a particular skill and our brain muscles and body are stimulated, like an expert – it is generally tested in the neuroscience field that if someone is sad and you are paying attention to them – your brain will mirror the sadness on their face. If you spend enough time with a sad person, then the chances are that you will become sad too.

Similarly, if you spend time with happy people, your brain will mirror their expression and action and your mood is likely to improve.

Mirror Neurons and Visualisation

David Hamilton explained that research studies on the mimic ability of mirror neurons show that when we hear a person speaking, our tongue muscles are also activated. The speaker in front of us though should have clarity in accent and voice. Similarly, if you have impaired movement and someone is describing that movement with clarity of voice and tone, you will notice that your ability to move would increase, and your brain map for that muscle would expand. You will soon notice that with an increased brain map, the area of your brain for those muscles will be expanded and you will start moving your muscle.

On the other hand, for wellness and wellbeing aspects of neuroplasticity, if we are sick and if we just listen and empathise with someone who talks about perfect health, then our mind will automatically start healing itself for wellbeing. But if we become sick in our society, people start drawing distances from patients and accuse them of their illness, reinforcing the sick mentality and inhibiting the brain's wellness response.

Mirror neuron activity increases if we simply *look* at someone's body parts. This in consequence increases the sensitivity of our own body parts. Alternatively, if we only *visualise* another person's body parts, then our own body parts become 'mirrored' and sensitised; the brain does not know the difference between real scenes we observe and imaginary scenes that we visualise.

If we *visualise* good health and optimistic thoughts, the appropriate chemicals are released and the right genes are activated or deactivated.

Ultimately, we become what we are imagining, so it is good to listen to someone live or via audio/video to get the benefit of positive imagining, to begin the healing processes in our mind. By instructed or guided imagery, we may heal any ache, pain or disease by looking, seeing, hearing and imagining.

Brain and Body Connections

Our brain is connected through our autonomic nervous system with eyes, lungs, liver, spleen, stomach, pancreas, intestines, kidneys, bladder, skin and reproductive organs. Our subconscious mind maintains all these systems unconsciously. That is why our belief, either conscious or subconscious, influences the systems and organs of the body.

When we expect something to happen, that happens at both the peripheral and autonomic nervous systems. Subsequently, it can be concluded that our thoughts can change the structure and function of our brain.

These thoughts send chemicals from the brain throughout our body. These chemical systems then interact with cells and even our genetic code. Research shows that if we focus on a part of our body, then the area of the brain that governs that part becomes activated, and that body part is also activated.

Affirmation

Affirmation means saying something repeatedly about our healing, wealth or happiness, because repetition tends to create neural connections in our brain. It generates more energy and neural connections become stronger. Then the mind triggers its journey to achieve that task. By repeatedly doing the following affirmations, we are able to improve our health, relationships, knowledge and wisdom. It is better to write down the affirmations and keep them in front of your mirror or study table or verbally say them to yourself 20 times in the morning and before retiring to bed so that with repeated exposure, your brain can begin to transform itself.

How to Safeguard your Plastic Mind from Negative Attitudes in Society?

In his book 'Magic of Thinking Big', David Schwartz suggests the following strategies to protect our minds from negativity. As we are the product of our environment, the association with negative people tends to make us think negatively. Close contact with petty individuals develops petty habits in us.

Companionship and association with people with big ideas raise the level of our thinking. Close contact with ambitious people gives us ambition; your personality, ambitions, present status in life, are all largely the result of your psychological environment. The person you will be next year, in five years, in the next ten years or twenty, will depend on your future environment. You change over months and years but how you will change depends upon your chosen environment.

Be Persistent to Achieve Your Goals

Successful people never surrender to suppressive

forces. People who never surrender are the happiest because they accomplish most. They find life stimulating and rewarding. They actively encounter other successful people each day, creating new opportunities via new ideas and new circumstances.

They make new friends, join new organisations, and enlarge their social orbit; variety in people and things add pleasure to life and gives it a broader dimension. They also select friends who have views different from themselves. Responsibilities and positions of high status precipitate individuals who are able to see both sides.

In the challenges of the 21st Century, narrow individuals do not have much of a future.

"Favour your subconscious mind."
When training your subconscious mind by affirmations and autosuggestions, this task and goal is achievable. You set the timeline for that goal. Your subconscious mind promptly starts working on that goal and brings you hundreds of

different solutions to achieve that goal.

Conversely, if you think about the goal and you consciously instigate negative autosuggestions to your mind, such as "I can't achieve this goal," then you may cause brain-procrastination. If you think and talk about that goal negatively, then your subconscious mind presents hundreds of reasons as to why this goal could not be achieved – *'As you sow, so shall you reap'*.

Chapter 9.

Music Therapies: Improve Neurodegenerative Diseases

9.1 Alzheimer's, Parkinson's and Autism

In her research paper, Monique Van Bruggen-Rufi defines and explains the history and role of music in neurodegenerative diseases as: "Music Therapy is the clinical and evidence-based interventions to accomplish certain goals within a therapeutic relationship by professional music therapists." She explained that "music therapies assess emotional wellbeing, physical health, social functioning, communication abilities and cognitive skills through musical responses."

Oliver Sacks, in his book, 'Musicophilia', explained that "listening to music is not just auditory and emotional, it is also a motoric activity – we listen to music with our muscles."

"Our faces and postures mirror the 'narrative' of the melody, and the thoughts and feelings it provokes."

Research on the effects of music on different neurological conditions is a new field of neurology. As music activates various regions of the brain, music can assist recovery in brain injuries and neurodegenerative diseases. Listening to music can alter brain structure and function, but the molecular mechanism behind these phenomena is still unknown.

A research study in Finland, by Chakravarthi Kanduri et al., 2015, has reported that "music listening can cause physiological changes in cerebral blood flow, cardiovascular muscle functioning and can also enhance dopamine secretion in the brain."

Music listening can regulate emotions and feelings of pleasure. Music is now being used as a therapeutic tool in clinical settings.

A systematic literature review published by Monique Van Bruggen-Rufi in 2015 in Netherlands, reported that, "... If we perform MRI to visualise the brain of music listeners, we will find that there are involvements in broad networks of the brain regions. Music listening can trigger the brain network in pre-frontal and interior frontal cortex, superior temporal poles and the cerebellum." And it was found that "if the music is emotionally meaningful to the listener, it activates the ventral tegmental area, the accumbens nucleus, and the hypothalamus."

It has been reported in this study that "there is a special relationship between music and motor neural circuits. It means that music can improve the movement problems of patients with Parkinson's disease and Huntington's disease." Music could activate the neural pathways in the brain regions like the insula, cingulate, cortex, hypothalamus, hippocampus, amygdala and pre-frontal cortex. These regions could be activated by music and provoke certain responses in these areas of the brain.

This research study performed by Monique Van Bruggen-Rufi suggests that patients with dementia, age-related conditions, developmental learning disabilities, addictions, brain injuries, physical disabilities or acute/chronic pain could benefit from this treatment. Music Therapies can target motor, cognitive, psychiatric, emotional and social disturbances.

9.2 Music Therapy can Treat Symptoms of Neurological Diseases

Lauren Banker defines Alzheimer's disease as "gradual neurodegenerative disease in which there is a formation of plaque growth, neuron decay and formation of neuro-fibrillary tangles throughout the brain, which causes cognitive behavioural and emotional deterioration, such as memory and language impairment."

Music therapy is one of the most cost-effective alternative therapies for Alzheimer's disease in which music is used to treat cognitive, behavioural and emotional symptoms. Music therapy is performed in two ways.

❖ Interactive Or Active
❖ Passive Or Receptive

Interactive or active therapy patients sing, hum, move along with music or play an instrument. In contrast, passive or receptive therapy patients only listen to live or recorded music and are less involved.

The following symptoms of Alzheimer's disease are improved by music therapy.

Improved Memory:

Music therapy greatly improves recalling old memories. When patients sing a familiar song, it enhances, recalls their date of birth and past memories. It also helps to form new memories. It means that music therapy acts as a catalyst to remembering old memories and forming new ones.

Improved Language Functioning and Communication:

Music therapy also improves language functioning and communications. Alzheimer's disease causes impaired language functioning. Patients with this disease cannot comprehend and produce language and have impaired judgement, and experience difficulty in expressing themselves.

When patients sing in therapy sessions, they are able to comprehend the topics of conversation better and stay focused on the topic more frequently.

They have increased communication and interaction with others, become socially more interactive, show improved greeting and complimenting behaviours and begin sharing jokes and memories.

Improved Behavioural Symptoms:

People living with Alzheimer's become more agitated when they experience difficulty in articulating their thoughts, needs or desires – music therapy helps them reduce agitated behaviours, including aimless wandering, verbal and physical aggression, repetitive sentences or questions and complaining. Patients who have been engaged in music therapy by *singing* and *playing* instruments exhibit reduced agitated behaviours.

Those who *listen* to music exhibit less agitated behaviours, become less insulting, are less attention-seeking, complaining and show a reduction in psychotic and psychological symptoms.

Improved Psychological Functioning:

Music therapy also improves psychological symptoms of Alzheimer's patients who have been exposed to *extended* therapy. It reduces symptoms of paranoia, hallucination and anxiety.

Improved Emotional Symptoms:

Music therapy has been effective in improving the emotional symptoms of Alzheimer's patients. Therapy reduces negative effects, such as stress. It also helps to elevate positive emotions and improve patients' mood.

After extensive music therapy, patients feel more positive and feel an increased sense of belonging and accomplishment.

9.3 Parkinson's Disease and Music Therapy

In Parkinson's disease, most patients suffer from the abnormality of voice and speech. Traditional pharmacological treatments and other speech therapies have not been particularly effective in treating these abnormalities. Consequently, 80% of people living with Parkinson's face difficulty speaking intelligibly, severely impairing their communication skills, and their ability to convey their emotional states and needs.

A comparative study by Catherine Y. Wan et al., in Harvard Medical School, reported that "an intensive voice therapy programme can be effective in minimising some of the speech abnormalities in patients with Parkinson's disease."

It is reported in the research studies that these improvements in speech abnormalities could be maintained even after 12 months of termination of treatment.

A research study shows that there is a significant improvement in vowel phonation and reading of the patients after 13 sessions of choral singing, which shows that singing could help improve speech-related complications and disorders in Parkinson's patients.

Music Therapy and Autism

Autism is a condition in which there is impairment in expression of language and communication. This condition affects about 1% of the population. Some autistic individuals have a lack of functional speech.

Music therapy helps improve this condition. Music intervention, designed to treat children with autism, is known as Auditory Motor Mapping Training (AMMT). This intervention involves three main components – singing, motor activity and imitation. This therapy engages the dysfunctional human mirror neuron system that is believed to be impaired in Autism. AMMT enhances the interaction between the auditory and motor systems, which is considered an effective therapy through which individuals with autism can develop their communication skills.

In Autism, the Impaired Language System is lateralised to the left hemisphere. Singing or intoned speaking engages a larger bi-hemispheric network. So when the words are sung, the phonemes are isolated, which are helpful in self-correction. Singing may help in engaging a brain network that facilitates sound motor mapping.

Music Therapy Alters Human Transcriptome

Chakravarthi Kanduri et al., 2015, studied the effect of listening to music on human transcriptome, reporting some significant changes in transcriptome of those who had actively participated in music therapy sessions.

Music has been an important part of cultural rituals in most societies. Nowadays, neurophysiological studies show that listening to or performing music has lasting effects on human brain structure and function. Listening to classical and soothing music has a profound effect on both body and brain. It regulates blood flow, improves heart and muscle functions and increases dopamine secretions in the human brain. Music evokes pleasure and regulates human emotions.

Other Practical Applications of Music Therapy

Arthur R. Pell, in his revised edition of Napoleon Hill's 'Think and grow Rich', explained the effect of music therapy applied to his young child born without any external or internal ear mechanisms. Pell explained that by applying music therapy, supported by his own *modus operandi* of faith and desire, he successfully recovered the hearing of his deaf and mute child. The child appeared to respond to the music therapy, and later, Pell decided the child needed further support and was instrumental in developing a suitable hearing aid in partnership with hearing aid companies.

He then did a lot of research and rendered his services to hearing aid instrument manufacturing companies for deaf and mute people.

Ancient Mystics Used Music Therapy to Heal

The ancient mystics were aware of the healing effects of music on body and mind. They used music therapy to heal many emotional disturbances. In modern times, we have music therapy, mantras and tuning forks to help adjust our behavioural and emotional issues.

Quantum physicists and mystics believe that "everything in the universe is made up of vibration frequencies."

Chapter 10.

Meditation & Mindfulness: Combat Neurodegenerative Diseases

"Trained Minds are psychologically different from Untrained Minds."

Meditation is a 'magical' drug for most mental and physical health conditions. Meditation can open your heart and mind to the wellbeing of yourself and those around you. Meditation concepts were brought to Western Societies by Eastern people and communities.

If you regularly practise meditation, it will bring profound positive effects to your mind, body, and soul. Meditation practice, if practised properly and regularly, will bring a chain of positive chemical reactions in your body; it will bring an inner balance in your life by strengthening intuition.

Meditation will connect your inner and outer

universal divine energy and bring balance and harmony with you and other people. Your self-esteem will go high; your attitude and vision toward life and people will change. By practising meditation, you transform from your past damaging and toxic thoughts to constructive future relationships and achievements.

These health and wellbeing qualities make meditation a therapeutic practice. It helps set new goals, aims and direction in your future life. Meditation greatly impacts the human brain; its end-results and benefits can be harnessed, and by properly practising it, you can enjoy the fruits of creativity, compassion, generosity, bliss and joy in life.

fMRI of results from trained and untrained meditated minds show profound differences in their structure and anatomy.

Naomi Ozaniec, in her book 'Beat Stress with Meditation' claims that "a correlation between mental activity and brainwave patterns has been known since the 1960s." Her findings have fuelled a cultural revolution that is centred on spiritualisation of values by introducing meditation principles of visualisation, relaxation and mindfulness techniques; according to Ozaniec, bio-feedback has moved to neuro-feedback.

Western objective laboratory technology and Eastern subjective experience technology have opened up the new era of 'Mind-Brain Interface Technology'.

The big questions of Western science and philosophy are whether 'Mind' is created by the brain, and whether consciousness itself might be reduced to neural activity. To answer these questions, Buddhism proposes a model that places the mind beyond the brain.

Meditation practises are regarded as beneficial to alter the structure and anatomy of the brain. Although meditation is a passive process, by involving loving, kindness and compassion practises, it brings both short-term and long-term neural changes.

Nowadays, by the application of fMRI, where Buddhist meditation meets Western technology and makes advancement in brain research, it is found that the brain has the capacity to develop new neural connections throughout life, which means that this neuroplasticity of the brain can make it possible to recover from injury and disease.

In a recent research report from the 'New York Academy of Sciences', Daniel A. Monti writes, "Meditation Techniques present a potential adjuvant treatment for patients with neurodegenerative diseases and are regarded as inexpensive and easy to teach and perform."

Meditation helps in improving cognition and memory in patients with neurodegenerative diseases. This review by Daniel A. Monti discusses the current data on meditation, memory and attention. It also describes the potential application of meditation in patients with neurodegenerative diseases.

Research by Rafal Marciniak et al., in 'Frontiers in Behavioural Neuro-Science' (2014), reported that many people suffer from Dementia, Alzheimer's and other Neurodegenerative Diseases, with ageing. The researchers pointed out that in the future there will be the need for appropriate therapy for these patients; based on both pharmacological and non-pharmacological interventions. They concluded that Meditation Techniques are one of the best possibilities of non-pharmacological interventions, which is now a subject of great scientific interest.

There are different categories of meditation based on the focus on single aspects, like breath or sounds. They are considered as 'Concentration-Meditation'.

Another category of meditation is based on aspiring to gain open attention, which contains more objects at once, or are selected in consecutive order. This category is based on awareness or open meditation. We can also divide meditation based on cognitive processes such as thought and images.

A third category is focused on your general mental development and cultivating a state of wellbeing, or it may be based on mental qualities like love, concentration or wisdom.

A review published by Alison in 2015 reported, "Meditation can change the size of key regions of our brain, improve our memory and make us more empathetic, compassionate and resilient under stress." According to this review, different meditation practices are receiving rising attention.

fMRI studies in various experiments show that meditation can be a beneficial and suitable non-pharmacological intervention to combat cognitive decline in the elderly. Meditation intervention improves the symptoms of Alzheimer's disease and cognition in the elderly. The other risk factors associated with Alzheimer's disease, such as hypertension, high cholesterol levels, poor cerebral blood flow, can be controlled by the impact of meditation on these patients.

An experiment by Rafal Marciniak et al., 2014, reported that 73 to 83-year-old elderly patients were randomly divided into three groups; the two based on different meditation techniques and a control group without any intervention. Patients given transcendental meditation and mindfulness meditation who performed it twice a day for 20 minutes at 12 weeks were transformed.

Furthermore, when the patients were examined and studied, the effect of meditation intervention was seen to improve cognitive flexibility, memory and verbal fluency after 18 months and then after 36 months. The results suggest that a strong improvement was in patients who used transcendental meditation, followed by mindfulness meditation, and the worst results were in control groups and in those that offered only relaxation programmes.

Even testing after three years showed 100% effects in persons using Transcendental meditation, and 87.5% effects were observed in those with Mindfulness Meditation Programmes. Similarly, another study to test the effect of Zen

Meditation on the decrease of grey matter thickness found that meditation increased the grey matter thickness in those who had Zen Meditation Intervention Therapy.

fMRI scans of meditating elderly patients show structural changes in several regions, such as an increased cortical thickness.

The most frequent changes reported are structural alterations in the anterior cingulate cortex superior, inferior frontal cortex and pre-frontal cortex. These regions are observed to be involved in attention and perceiving internal sensory processes and cognitive functions. Some studies have reported an increased volume of the hippocampus that is important for memory.

10.1 Meditation is the 'Fountain of Youth'

Meditation increases brain grey matter and optimises brain functioning – those who meditate purposefully can achieve a new state of consciousness and become successful in improving their mental and physical health.

116

Skilful and productive meditation requires conscious practised effort.

Meditation can improve concentration and intelligence, and it lessens anxiety and depression. You can experiment with the different meditation methods available to choose the one that is the most appropriate for you.

- ❖ *'Concentration-based Meditation'* will improve your concentration.
- ❖ *'Mindful Meditation'* will improve your mood.

Meditation can be practised several times daily, once a day, weekly or even monthly. However, most experts recommend you meditate every day for 10-30 minutes to acquire the maximum benefit. Incorporating meditation into your everyday life is recommended for re-balancing the body.

10.2 Chemistry of the Meditating Brain

Serotonin: Meditation boosts serotonin, which is

117

a mood-controlling neurotransmitter.

Cortisol: Meditation neutralises cortisol, which is a major age-accelerating hormone. When stressed, our body produces a lot of cortisol and adrenaline, which leads to anxiety, depression, increased blood pressure, brain fog, insomnia and inflammation. Mindfulness meditation reduces cortisol.

Dehydroepiandrosterone (DHEA) is a life-longevity molecule and is the most important hormone in the body. As we get older, our DHEA levels decrease year after year. Low levels make us more susceptible to diseases and accelerate ageing. By measuring DHEA levels, we can estimate physiological 'true age'. The lower your DHEA level is, the fewer years you have left. However, meditation provides a dramatic boost to DHEA hormone levels. Meditation practitioners have 43.7% more DHEA than anyone else.

Gamma-aminobutyric Acid (GABA) makes you feel calm. Alcohol, drugs, tobacco and caffeine addictions reduce the levels of GABA in the body.

Lack of GABA can cause anxiety, nervousness, racing heart and sleeplessness. It is found that levels of GABA increase by 27% after 60 minutes of mindfulness meditation.

Endorphin: Meditation boosts endorphin levels. It is the hormone of happiness. It is produced in the body, and it is used as an internal painkiller. After long-distance running, endorphins rush into the body, resulting in a heightened sense of wellbeing; that is why many runners are 'addicted' to their sport. The good news is that this wonderful state of mind can be achieved through meditation.

Growth Hormone (GH) is released during meditation, which simultaneously boosts GH. High levels of GH are produced during childhood, sustained in the body until you enter into your 40's when growth hormone begins to decrease. Depletion of GH from the body causes weaker bones and muscles, poor heart contractions, mood swings, lack of motivation, fatigue and increases body fat. Growth hormones are also released during the deepest state of sleep, called the *delta state*. That is why meditators generally look young and healthy.

Growth hormones are produced in our pituitary gland, which is situated at the base of the brain.

Melatonin levels in the body are also boosted through meditation. Produced by the pineal gland, its level in the blood increases throughout waking hours and is at its peak just before going to sleep. Meditation practitioners have 98% increases in melatonin levels. Melatonin strengthens the immune system, slows down ageing, and prevents cancer. It is thought to be linked to the prevention of over 100 different diseases, and is a key to good mood and restful sleep.

Mindfulness can Heal Neurological Diseases and Disorders

Dr Jessamy Hibberd and Jo Usmar, in their book 'Make you Mindful', define Mindfulness as 'a practise of awareness'. It is a technique for learning to become more aware of your thoughts, emotions, body, impulses, urges and the world around you. Mindfulness is a brilliant way of getting to know oneself better.

Mindfulness is not a quick fix. It is a skill that you have to learn like any other, e.g., cooking, playing games, drawing and skiing. Mindfulness requires time to learn and practise and also energy. If you stick with it – you will get lots of rewards.

After practising it, you will find yourself more engaged with life. You will find yourself more present in everything you do. If you have thoughts and doubts in your mind about your future and past issues that are left unresolved, mindfulness will make your life happier, exciting and wonderful – you will be able to deal with upsetting or stressful things.

Marchand, W. R. (2011) reported in 'World Journal of Radiology' that "Mindfulness practise is the moment-by-moment awareness of sensations, emotions and thoughts… Mindfulness-based interventions are used for stress, psychological wellbeing, coping with chronic illness and are used as adjunctive treatments for psychiatric disorders; but the neural mechanism associated with mindfulness has not yet been well characterised."

fMRI studies show that mindfulness impacts the function of the pre-frontal medial cortex, insula and amygdala. Mindfulness practice affects lateral frontal regions, basal ganglia and the hippocampus.

Zeidan. F, in 2014, reported in the review 'Neuro-biology of Mindfulness' that *Mindful Meditation* can improve a range of mental and physical health problems. He has reported that neuro-imaging is beginning to identify the brain mechanisms that mediate the relationships between mindfulness, meditations and the results obtained by such interventions. Mindfulness meditations can result in the enhancement in sensory awareness, cognition; hence, health and wellbeing can be accomplished through meditation practise.

Chapter 11.
Metacognition And
Executive Brain Functions

"Role of metacognition in mind healing,
empowerment and creativity"

Cognition means acquiring knowledge and information for learning thinking and creating wisdom.

Metacognition is the ability to think beyond cognition or cognition about cognition or thinking about thinking and knowing about knowing, which means awareness about awareness. In other words, metacognition is knowing about the mysteries of the mind and how it acquires awareness, consciousness, and thinking. Such a skill is the higher-order thinking or metacognition and is acquired and used to reach the level of transcendental genius level of consciousness. Understanding and knowing about all these mechanisms of the mind could benefit individuals and societies to acquire an out of box thinking. Such a mind could take societies and civilisations

123

out beyond the boundaries of ignorance.

The term metacognition was first coined by American Psychologist John H. Flavell, who defined the concept as, "Knowledge about functioning of cognition and to take control of the cognitive process in the human brain."

In the domain of cognitive neuroscience, the metacognitive skills have the greatest role in the development and growth of the prefrontal cortex, which is the CEO of the brain and is responsible for all types of mental organisation, command, planning and delivering tasks and duties to all other parts of the brain. The functions that program the brain by goal settings, task completion and giving direction towards mission and passion facilitate the growth of prefrontal cortex. This makes the brain smarter and focused, optimises its achievements and maximises its function and capacity. The metacognitive theory indicates that we can change our attitude and behaviour by giving a higher frequency of positive thoughts to our mind and body, usually by sticking to the self-help and positive psychology.

This improves the frequency of positive thoughts, which ultimately impact greatly our overall mental well-being, success, and ultimate happiness. This is because the brain gets more growth with positive and optimistic thoughts rather than judging things and people with a negative point of view.

For example, if we believe that using less fuel and electricity will reduce the gas and electricity bill, on the other hand, it will also save the planet from being more polluted with heat and gases; similarly, quitting smoking will save our health, money and also protect others from getting negatively impacted by passive smoking. On the other hand, this too will protect our environment and planet. The global artwork is one of the best types of metacognitive training and knowledge. Our mind perceives from the artifact of global art, music and literature (book novel and fiction industry). By training our mind with metacognitive abilities, we can bring back the wandering mind to more worthwhile tasks rather than (wondering) using our mental capacities in non-productive and worthless ways.

Applying metacognitive strategies in schools and developing metacognitive abilities in young students will enable them to learn more and have clarity in thinking.

11.1 Transcendental and Metacognitive Brain

Why are Metacognitive Brains More Stable than Cognitively-Aware or Scholarly Brains?

The difference between the cognitive and metacognitive brain is that the metacognitive brain is more stable, functional, and creative.

Research paper, "The Triangle of Spirituality Intelligence Metacognition and Consciousness," published by Athanasios Drigas and Eleni Mitsea, described that the scientific community recognises spirituality as a fundamental factor of human intelligence in the history of human beings. Researchers from diverse fields of knowledge such as psychology, medicine, educational sciences, economy and business management have recognised the notion of spiritual intelligence as one of the most controversial and highly debated notions. The result of this research study shows that spiritual intelligence is the backbone of every other human intelligence. Spiritual intelligence integrates and transforms every physical, intellectual and emotional ability from self-awareness and self-knowledge to higher consciousness.

Our metacognitive abilities and executive functions in our brain develop and mature when we are able to organise our knowledge at a hierarchical level.

At a higher level of thinking metacognitively or at a transcendental genius level, one could develop the habits and norms of self-observation and self-regulation by giving attention to our emotions and impulses to our inward reality. So, by this inward attention, we could become capable of controlling our emotions and impulses.

By this inward attention or higher-order thinking on our true self, we can focus our attention toward our real problems and make our mind a problem solver and the world a worth living place. Life becomes easier for us consequently, which gives us mental flexibility, stability and optimisation to our external environment.

It is a well-known fact that intelligence is the only factor, which contributes in neuroplasticity or brain development; in western culture, mysteries about the historical development of knowledge and mental healing by meditation were brought in and introduced by eastern cultures and their mystics. In most of the eastern traditions, it was thought that spiritual mysteries have the ultimate answer for the nature of knowledge, intelligence and consciousness.

World-renowned psychologists such as Abraham Maslow, Carl Jung, Raymond D. Fowle, Carl Ransom Rogers have mentioned in their theories that spirituality plays an important role in the development of human personality; in most studies, it was found that spiritual intelligence is the superior and more integrative form of intelligence that is blended or acquired by the proper development of our thinking mechanism.

By letting go of our desires after attachment with

128

it could harness and leverage the success in our life. The other spiritual way to attract desires and successes is to know about our life problems and purposes from the deepest sources; which means going deep into the real meaning and purpose of life. Understanding the purpose of life and the universe itself will broaden our mind and enhance our cognition to the metacognitive level, which is an intrinsic characteristic of the sophisticated, smarter and universal mind.

So, being enlightened means being more prosperous and healthier rather than remaining obscure or ignorant. It means seeing deeper into the illusions of the world and universe. Because seeing the world from a superficial level is nothing more than an illusion. Looking and feeling it by deeper senses or sixth senses or by intuition and meditation and feeling its musical signals coming to us through vibrations from subatomic strings in the universe, that is real.

All golden treasures of spirituality, goodness, wealth, happiness and prosperity are not lying on the surface or illusion but are a little bit deeper and submerged into the intellect, wisdom, nobility, understanding, harmony, coherency and creativity; so by knowing or understanding the purpose of life, most importantly health, wealth and happiness bring you all happiness, wealth and good health. Gradually with our own speed and understanding, we will know about the meaning and purpose of life and the universe. The role of spiritual intelligence or transcendentalism is uplifting our cognitive sense to the metacognitive or superconscious level.

Maslow Psychology and Self-Transcendence

According to Maslow, self-transcendence is self-motivation and is beyond self-actualisation. According to him, transcendence is the highest and most holistic level of human consciousness. This includes a good relationship with other human beings, other animal species, and being friendly to other nations, civilisations, and the cosmos. A transcendent person seeks something beyond personal benefit; they strive to advance and further science, art and spirituality for great causes, like the cause of serving others. They expand their identification beyond the personal ego.

A transcendent person experiences awareness of their human potential and they feel alive in a world that overflows with truth and beauty. They speak the language of unity and eternity. When two transcendents meet each other, they can recognise each other even upon the first meeting and can instantly come into harmony with each other and mutual understanding. Transcendents are holistic and they have natural cooperation in differentiating between selfishness and unselfishness. They can easily control and go beyond their emotions or ego and self-identity.

By being transcendent, our vision gets illuminated and clearer, leading us to have a bigger brain and a bigger heart that accommodates a lot of knowledge and wisdom within us. This accumulation and accommodation of a bigger structure of knowledge within us will lead us to discoveries and innovations.

Walsh and Vanshan, in their research on

spirituality, claim that transcendents have capabilities of expansion of our consciousness by application of art preserved in the core of societies. These qualities in transcendentalists could purify human-distorted emotions and scattered desires into a stable personality. There are three different elements of transcendentalism that encompass the world's greatest religious traditions and help individuals purify from emotional and attentional instabilities.

Ethics

Ethics or positive attitude and optimism in life protect and save us from greed and anger, and cultivate kindness, compassion and calmness in our life.

Attentional Training

By training our minds to retain and sustain our brain's memory system to advance our perceptions by broader reading, observations and experimentations and by learning various skills and arts by hit and trial methods would improve our focus and attention systems in our brains. This would ultimately regulate our emotions, moods and behaviours and make us more motivated, ambitious, passionate and mission-oriented individual in societies. So, overcoming this wandering state of mind by improving our focus could make us more productive and conscious.

Emotional Transformations

We should first be aware of any kind of destructive emotions like fear, anger and prejudice in our heart, mind and soul. Then, we should take special measures to stabilise our minds toward advancement and education of our emotions with techniques of focus, attention and uplifting of our memory system by observations, experimentation and reading techniques to regulate our emotions. We should also channel positive attitudes by reading good psychology books to cultivate positivity in our system and eliminate any inherited negative flood of emotions in our daily lives through media; including TV, newspapers, and other negativity around society. We should cultivate and harness equanimity, which means keep up our self-calm and focus during fear, storm and unfavorable conditions. But we should learn how to be creative and to stay calm in unfavourable situations in our life.

The person harbouring the mind of a transcendent should be able to control his self-oriented personality to an allocentric personality, becoming a person with greater communal and societal interests at heart. A transcendent person believes that keeping attention on the present moment will open our inner eye.

Due to fully practising spiritual intelligence, transcendental minds could attain final unity in the path of human evolution for consciousness. If we keep waking up our consciousness while ageing we could develop our personality through applying skills of spiritual intelligence. With spiritual intelligence, we feel unity and oneness with others. According to Plotinus, "The full reality of self is only possible by mystical awakening and awareness."

Role of Spiritual Intelligence in Metacognitive Level of Consciousness

Metacognition is the ability or cognition process that makes us self-actualise and regulate our emotional processes towards achieving goals and missions. The purpose of metacognition and spiritual intelligence is to actualise our potential to expand our self-consciousness and awareness of our existence, including self-perception, self-experience and self-control. Metacognition could keep make us learn from our experiences to become aware of our thoughts, to have clear concept of our real identity, which could improve our brain plasticity, awareness, self-regulation, which in return could help us develop self-control skills of attention, stress management, impulse and emotions such as anger. Metacognition could also help us improve our attention and memory by applying the methods of metacognition that play an important role in our spiritual development.

Brain research shows that during meditation, the brain increases its growth in frontal areas due to focus and improved attention, due to which the metacognitive state of a stable mind is achieved. The development of spiritual intelligence in today's societies is the most demanded methodology for improving and developing physical and mental health in any work environment, businesses, daily life, and successful leaderships. Spiritual intelligence could create and promote better leaders and peacemakers and innovators of coming centuries.

According to T.S Elliot, spiritual intelligence is the pathway to the knowledge that we have lost and will lose in the flood of information around us in the form of global internet and artificial intelligence. We have lost the taste of life in running for better living and we have lost our wisdom and passion in learning of non-creative and non-productive knowledge, which has a negative impact on the development and propagation of our wisdom, nobility and honesty or higher-order thinking as well as in the development of our executive brain functions like goal settings or brain planning and organisation. The great polymath philosopher Benjamin

Franklin would always keep his diary of goals and aims, which helped him bring his emotions and nerve impulses under the command of logic and reasoning. This metacognitive ability to manage his nerves and emotions had always placed him on a higher level of intelligence and made him a highly influenced person in the history of mankind.

A recent neuroscience research shows that those who have acquired this metacognitive ability in their life had more gray matter in the anterior prefrontal cortex of their brain. The growth in the prefrontal cortex in human brain due to executive brain functions, goal settings and organisation have made human beings more intelligent, civilised and unique on this planet. Executive functions are those cognitive skills that are used to control and coordinate our other cognitive abilities and behaviours.

The executive functions' deficiency in the brain causes damage to the frontal lobe and parietal lobes. The frontal lobes are the last areas of the brain to develop in the evolution of man. This area of the brain develops very late in human beings than in the primate. It covers 40% of the human brain. When the executive brain function system is damaged, we could face the following impairment in our brain functions.

1.   Difficulty in organising our goals, aims, life and mission and purpose in life.

2.   Mood swings and a lack of interest in people and other life around us.

3.   Inappropriate behaviour and a lack of understanding from past actions.

According to the research published in the department of medical psychology journal in Hamburg University Germany, the metacognitive interventions were studied in patients suffering from anxiety, obsessive compulsive disorders, social anxiety disorders, post-traumatic stress disorders, depression and schizophrenia, chronic fatigue syndrome, body dysmorphic disorders, emotional instabilities, alcohol addiction, sexual disorder, eating disorder and personality disorders. These metacognitive interventions in large groups of patients with various conditions have been found very effective and promising.

11.2 Self Actualisation

Self-actualisation is the complete realisation of one's potential and the full development of one's abilities and appreciation for life. Self-actualisation emerges when more basic needs are met. These are already well-accepted people of society. They have common abilities to cultivate deep loving relationships. Self-actualisation could also be called self-realisation or self-cultivation.

Abraham Maslow was the original founder of the term self-actualisation. Self-actualisation is the ultimate goal of every organism and is referred to as the main desire of self-fulfilment. Every animal and plants have an inborn soul of self-actualisation. If an individual is fully functional, they have moved toward the process of inward knowing or are increasingly listening to their deepest psychological and emotional being. They have attained a greater accuracy and true self.

Fully functional people are in touch with their feelings and abilities. They are able to trust their innermost urges and intuitions.

Chapter 12.

Brain Waves, Mind Healing And Creativity

Creativity and good mental health are the matter of having right brain waves. When creative people are in an imaginative state, they experience alpha brain waves. Alpha brain waves are more creative. Tony Robbins says, "There is no problem that cannot be solved in alpha."

Well-trained brains with alpha brain waves have 50% increase in creativity. A research study was conducted by Doctor James V Hardt in Stanford Research Institute. Volunteers of the study were given creative tasks before and after the alpha waves training. Profound increase in 50% of creativity was noted in all individuals receiving these alpha waves. Some of them successfully solved the academic and social problems with which they were struggling for over two years.

When your brain is in high alpha state, it assembles information from the knowledge hidden in your body's cellular and subconscious system that you may have forgotten in the routine of daily life. But the data of that knowledge may have been stored in your subconscious mind during the course of certain life experiences. To address life's hard problems in such a creative way by getting alpha brain training will make you a unique creative person possessing highly creative abilities.

Highly creative people have profound ability to train their brain to an alpha state to attain the solutions of problems in their life as well as of societies. Highly creative people are always experiencing a boosted alpha state of their minds.

In research studies, individuals receiving the boosted alpha waves were found to be more creative and better problem solvers than those who had ignored and were untrained to reach the alpha state of mind. EOC institute website published the findings about the impact of brain waves on the creativity of brains. According to these findings, nerve cells of our brains fire electrical signals all the time, which results in a specific brain wave pattern. These highly unique patterns of brain waves are connected to our thoughts, emotions, biological chemistry and all other things relevant to consciousness.

One can improve their alpha brain state by following the beats and brain waves set up in the EquiSync sound technology, which is a trademarked brand for audio patterns containing brain neural beats. These are sold in the form of audio CD's which were created by Robert Monroe as a HemiSync technology specifically for synchronisation of brain hemispheres. According to Monroe, these technologies can synchronise the two hemispheres of the brain and are used for many purposes including relaxation, sleep induction, learning, memorisation. It also helps to cope with physical and mental difficulties and helps to reach the altered state of consciousness. Monroe has claimed that listening to them by using headphones could trigger various brain waves activities in your brain and you can feel various states of brain waves including alpha, beta, gamma and theta brain waves.

Robert Allen Monroe was born on October 30,

1915 in Indiana and died on March 17, 1995 at an age of 79. He did his BA from Ohio State University. Professionally, he was a radio broadcaster. He specialised in psychology medicine, biodentistry, psychiatry, electrical engineering, physics and education. He developed this HemiSync technology that facilitates and enhances brain performance. Following different types of brain waves could be triggered into your brain by this HemiSync technology.

13.1 Alpha Waves: Waves Between 7-13 Hz

When you have alpha waves in your brain during meditative state or musical state or when your brain is receiving a boosted dose of alpha waves by listening to HemiSync audios, you will start creating the ideas and thoughts mostly in the form of alpha waves. This is the state of brain when you receive alpha waves sitting calmly and alone in a relaxing manner and waiting for ideas to grace your brain. When you receive one good idea in your mind while sitting calmly, you will suddenly experience a traffic of great ideas starting to flow into your mind. Nothing physically happens in your brain, instead it is the circuit of alpha brain waves passing through the track of your brain usually called brain motor, which is similar to a device or motor constructed to calculate electric current passing through it.

Calmly sitting in your room, anywhere in countryside or near a lake or in a jungle with a pen and paper handy to record and write your thoughts, you will find your brain performance enhanced soon. Then, in less than one year you will have developed great writing skill, ability to think clearly, talk more efficiently and to plan for your financial life and career. More importantly, you will soon start getting closer to the ultimate realities of life, the purpose of life, universe, and most importantly, the nature and composition of spirit and spirituality.

Last but not the least, you will learn how to succeed in life and start living the life of high achiever. Further, you can become a great creator, innovator and builder of personalities, nations and global communities and a dream civilisation by Alpha waves generation in your brain.

Following these practices, you will keep your body away from gaining weight, anxiety, stress and hopelessness, and keeping healthy balance in the creative and pleasure centres of your brain.

The other important benefits of acquiring the state of alpha waves through these meditation techniques are:

- Ability to read books calmly and silently
- Listening to and enjoying music
- Writing your short term and long-term goals and reviewing them regularly
- Becoming a comedian then a serious actor within your intrinsic wisdom system. Your life will be full of fun rather than misery
- Your parasympathetic system will start avoiding social and spiritual sins to maintain a healthy balance between itself and your synthetic nervous system.

When you have a negative parasympathetic nervous system, you will become more immune to diseases and sicknesses and become overweight or overburdened with sin or immorality, which is

146

not good for your overall body homeostasis, circulation, excretion and digestion, respiration and skin health.

Other Significant Benefits of Meditating Using Aforementioned Methods

Meditation upgrades a key brain region by boosting alpha waves in it. You feel less stress, more happiness, more success, deep sleep, easier learning, better memory, higher IQ and EQ. You can change your brain and your life through meditation.

Meditation balances your left and right brain hemispheres, which results in overall brain synchronisation. This harmony and synchronisation in both brain parts will make you a fast learner, with good mental and physical health, great creativity and a productive mind. That's why meditators usually look decades younger than their actual age; they also live a longer life. Practising meditation will make you more creative and innovative.

Meditation boosts your body chemicals like

endorphins and serotonin, which are essential neurotransmitters for creativity and art production. While meditation lowers stress hormones like cortisol and adrenaline, it has many benefits of bringing natural pleasure, happiness and contentment through creativity. Creators, innovators and productive thinkers live better, healthier and more content life than non-creative people.

Meditation has a great impact on gut brain to transform your microbiome into probiotics, which will ultimately facilitate the brain to work more efficiently. Meditation can make bodies of meditators very slim, pruned and so helps them maintain their ideal body posture. Powerful CEOs, famous Hollywood actors, bestselling authors, well-known media personalities, professional athletes and billionaires have revealed that the secret of their success lies in meditation, and they practise it regularly in their life.

Meditation heals your body at the cellular level, because some 50 trillion body cells come in harmony with each other in a meditative state.

The people who have long history of suffering, failure and distraction have achieved their dreams and success in life when they started meditation to pursue their objectives and goals in life. Meditation has a great potential to kick-start your neurogenesis to develop a neuroplastic brain with a bigger frontal cortex and a smart brain with organised executive brain functions and goal settings. Meditative brain learns creativity, and creativity leads to books, movies, songs, technology and inventions in societies.

Intuition is the source of all scientific, literary, artistic wisdom and was the real way of Einstein's creativity and his greatest theory of relativity. Similarly, it was the source of wealth for Warren Buffett, Bill Gates and Elon Musk. Intuition is the result of meditative practices that enhance this ability in our brain and boosts creativity.

Conclusion

Neuroscience of Mind Empowerment is a part of the Neurocosmic Project for Global Enlightenment, Consciousness and Creative Culture.

The contents of this innovative and abundant model are based on the following therapeutic, metacognitive, and creative approaches for mind healing, metacognition, and creativity.

Goal Settings and Executive Brain Function

Proper planning your imaginations make you a fortunate being. We can make our pre-frontal cortex and Hippocampus smarter by setting short term and long-term goals to reach the targets of our life missions and passions, and to develop the vision of professionals and legends. We should keep on moving forward in our career or missionary life with developing our executive brain functions by managing our pre-frontal cortex by these high achievements' tools in our life. A conspicuous growth of grey matter in the brain could be seen by fMRI scans of a person following written goals and aims in his or her life. This on-going daily growth with goals routines in life will make the life of a person longer, smarter, and more successful than those who are randomly following life purposes without written goals. Such a purposeful person with missionary life will be happier and more satisfied due to harnessing the more honesty pure wisdom which is golden treasure of happiness, contentment, and great wealth by gaining the trust of societies and humanity at large.

On the other hand, empathy, honesty, and wisdom are essential elements and ingredients to make your soul free from psychosomatic illness and social sins e.g., anger, envy, jealousy, and revenge which are negative emotions that are a natural part of the human soul.

"Sometimes your honesty makes other people honest with you."

This is an out of box thinking and most effective way of leadership and prolonging your ruling and kingdom in any field of life. Clinically, it is the best approved attitude of making your body immune from illness and infections. On one hand, it is a faith, and on the other, it is the placebo effect, on which modern clinical psychology and pathology are based. Adapting such positive and optimistic attitudes, always viewing, and visualizing positive results, will produce and attract more success than expecting negativity and failure which unfortunately is widespread in our societies.

ADAPTING LIFESTYLE ACCORDING TO EPIGENETICS RULES CAN ENHANCE YOUR NEUROPLASTICITY AND MIND POWER

Fueling our minds with positive thoughts, high dimensional knowledges, and a conducive environment for living will make our minds and bodies like a spiritual machine predicting and creating the knowledges of ultimate truths and realities of the universe from its intrinsic body system and outer environment. This is because human bodies contain at a subatomic level the whole universe, even subatomic particles and most of the basic chemicals from other galaxies. You will dig deeper into your intrinsic body system

152

through meditation and other therapies discussed in the book, including organization of complex knowledge structure either manually or electronically. By practicing these methods and knowledge, the DNA of your body will start unfolding and expressing itself and will gradually start raising your intelligence, consciousness, and other wisdoms. Silent and dormant genes will start expressing your cellular memory and other neural systems memories like solar plexus, heart, and gut. The brain will start getting conscious until you reach the highest level of super-genius consciousness.

A person with such a consciousness and enlightenment will have a broader vision toward life, societies, and the universe. In this way, you can overcome your fears due to ignorance, diseases, and environmental disasters of weathers, volcanos, oceans, and other universal disasters due to meteorites collisions with planet earth, satellites, and spaceships debris around the earth, overheating of the sun due to stars collisions, black holes formations due to novas and supernovas.

By carefully exploring vital regions of the brain, the author of the book firmly believes that human brains' vital organs are thrusting and hungry for getting their full nourishment from this universal knowledge and wisdom of art, music, and spirituality. Every human could be able to get this vital fuel, which is the common heritage of humanity to acquire full consciousness, the malleable mind prone to change itself according to wisdom. On the other hand, DNA is also prone to mutations relative to its good environment and consciousness.

Global democratization of science education system and spirituality would be of great help to citizens of countries to get benefit from these universal sources of knowledges.

The establishment of creative institutes and industries in the form of fiction and non-fiction book industries and converting the stories of these books into their graphic form, film, or in art and sculpture form will educate the human brain to understand following the emotions of his or her fellow human properly and logically. These industries could better educate the emotions of citizens and nations and will make them humbler and more humane with fellow citizens, with nature, and with the universe. It is a universal fact that today's economically and culturally prosperous countries and nations are the result of quality creative products from these knowledge economies. These products have a great global market where other developed countries can trade their books, films, music, sports, research on spirituality and other cultural shows to harmonize the global communities.

In local markets, the products from these industries could propel the growth of creativity and innovation and productivity which is an engine of prosperity. But those countries and their heads of states who are reluctant to develop these knowledge-based economies in their states, it is speculated that in coming decades the brain growth and intelligence geniuses or those intellectual who are main power of this economy including scientists, philosophers, artists, writers, poets, and musicians will perish from those nations. All other states lacking this intelligence and wisdom will desperately become dependent on states enriched in these industries and creative culture. They must follow their economical and foreign policies. Ultimately brains from these regions will start shrinking and become extinct like many plants and animal species are at high risks of extinction due to severe inevitable environmental factors of drought and famine in these areas.

So, to keep on flourishing the terrestrial brain, we must tackle these challenges and problems. This vital human organ is facing extinction globally and specifically in Africa, Asia, Latin America, East and Middle East, and other regions of the globe, where brain health and growth is severely ignored due to environmental and cultural challenges.

Glossary

Abundance: a great, plentiful amount, an overflowing fullness, ample sufficiency, profusion, copious supply, superfluity of wealth – in the context of this book, it is more than merely material wealth or possessions.

Accumbens: the nucleus accumbens (NAc) is a key brain region mediating a variety of behaviours, including reward and satisfaction, addiction, the regulation of emotions induced by music, and its connected role in mediating dopamine release. The NAc has a role in rhythmic timing and is considered to be of central importance to the limbic-motor interface. Significantly, in July 2007, Jon-Kar Zubieta published findings that the NAc is central to the machinery of the placebo effect. This confirmed that specific neural circuits and neurotransmitter systems respond to the expectation of benefit during placebo administration and that these expectations induce measurable physiological changes.

Affluence: having a great amount of monetary wealth, land and/or an unfettered beneficiary of scarce resources.

Amygdala: an almond-shaped mass of nuclei (cells) located deep within both temporal lobes of the brain. There are two amygdalae, one in each brain hemisphere. The amygdala is a limbic system structure involved in many of our emotions and motivations, particularly those related to survival; processing emotions such as fear, anger and pleasure.

Articulated: able to express thoughts and feelings easily and clearly or showing this quality.

Autism: is part of a range of conditions known as Autistic Spectrum Disorders (ASD) that affect the way the brain processes information. Autism is a developmental disorder that can cause problems with social interaction, language skills and physical behaviour, and the world can appear chaotic with no clear boundaries, order or meaning. The disorder varies from mild to so severe that sufferers may almost be unable to communicate and need round-the-clock care.

Basal Ganglia: a group of nuclei (clusters of neurons) in the brain that are located deep beneath the cerebral cortex (the highly convoluted outer layer of the brain). Basal ganglia specialise in processing information on movement and in fine-tuning the activity of brain circuits that determine the best possible response in a given situation (e.g., using the hands to catch a ball or using the feet to run). Thus, they play an important role in planning actions required to achieve a particular goal, executing well-practised habitual actions, and learning new actions in novel situations.

Bliss: delight, ecstasy, euphoria, rapture, gladness, blessedness, joy, exaltation, satisfaction, pleasure, happiness, paradise – the opposite of distress, grief, woe, misery, anguish, unhappiness, heartbreak and wretchedness.

Cerebellum: the part of the brain located in the posterior cranial fossa behind the brainstem. It consists of two cerebellar lobes and a middle section called the vermis. Three pairs of peduncles link it with the brainstem. Its functions are concerned with coordinating voluntary muscular activity.

Cerebral Cortex: a thin mantle of grey matter covering the surface of each cerebral hemisphere. The cerebral cortex is crumpled and folded, forming numerous convolutions (gyri) and crevices (sulci). It is made up of six layers of nerve cells and the nerve pathways that connect them. The cerebral cortex is responsible for the processes of thought, perception, and memory and serves as the seat of advanced motor function, social abilities, language, and problem-solving.

Cingulate Cortex: a component of the limbic system of the brain, responsible for producing emotional responses to physical sensations of pain.

Cognitive: relating to mental processes concerned with knowledge, perception, memory, judgment and reasoning, as contrasted with emotional and volitional processes, etc.

COMT-Gene provides instructions for making and maintains appropriate levels of the enzyme, catechol-O-methyltransferase. It is particularly important in the brain's pre-frontal cortex, which is involved with personality, planning, inhibition of behaviours, abstract thinking, emotion and working (short-term) memory, organising and coordinating information from other parts of the brain.

Comprehended: understand the nature or meaning of; grasp with the mind; perceive.

Consciousness: a complex concept, one that includes memory, cognition, input from the senses, and an awareness of selfhood; essentially, the cognition of one's self, one's past, and one's potential futures, and the relationship between the mind and the physical world, at any given moment.

Delta state (of sleep): one of 5 different wavelengths that function in the brain – alpha, beta, *delta*, gamma, and theta. In our deepest sleep state, delta brain waves are dominant. Delta waves are the *slowest* recorded brain waves in human beings. They are found most often in infants and young children. As we age, we tend to produce fewer delta brain waves, even during deep sleep. Delta waves are associated with the deepest levels of relaxation and restorative, healing sleep. Adequate production of delta waves helps us feel rejuvenated after a good sleep. If there is abnormal delta activity, an individual may experience learning disabilities or have difficulties maintaining conscious awareness (such as in cases of brain injuries).

Dementia: not a disease in itself, but a progressive disorder; a group of symptoms that may accompany a number of diseases that affects the brain, particularly the ability to remember, think and reason. The most common of these is Alzheimer's disease. Another is vascular dementia which can develop following a stroke or blood vessel damage that interrupts the flow of blood to the brain. Dementia is not a consequence of growing old but the risk of having dementia increases with age.

Dissuaded: to prevent someone from a purpose or course of action by persuasion.

Dopamine: a neurotransmitter produced by the brain, having several different functions, playing a critical role in the function of the central nervous system. It is also linked with the brain's complex system of motivation and reward. Altered levels of this neurotransmitter in the brain can cause a range of symptoms and problems, ranging from Parkinson's disease to Attention Deficit Disorder (ADD). In Parkinson's, low dopamine levels make patients shaky, weak, and confused, with impaired control over their bodies.

Eating Disorders: characterised by an abnormal attitude towards food that causes someone to change their eating habits and behaviour, leading them to make unhealthy choices about food with damaging results to their health. E.g. *anorexia nervosa* – when a person tries to keep their weight as low as possible by starving themselves and/or exercising excessively. *Bulimia* – when a person goes through periods of binge eating and then makes themselves deliberately vomit or uses laxatives to try to control their weight.

Endorphins: our natural pain and stress fighters, endorphins are among the brain chemicals known as neurotransmitters, which help transmit electrical signals within the nervous system. At least 20 types of endorphins have been demonstrated in humans. They interact with the opiate receptors in the brain to reduce our perception of pain and act similarly to drugs such as morphine and codeine.

Emotional Intelligence: a description of how well an individual is able to be in touch with their feelings and sense how those around them are feeling to determine the best course of action when a choice must be made. It is not an inherent skill; anyone can learn, develop and apply it. Potentially dangerous situations can develop if people use their emotional intelligence in a way that benefits them only. By understanding the core emotions of those around us, and the negatives can be balanced properly, emotional intelligence will always be important.

Epigenetics: study of potentially heritable changes in gene expression (active versus inactive genes) that does not involve changes to the underlying DNA sequence – which in turn affects how cells read the genes. Epigenetic change is regular and natural but can also be influenced by factors including age, the environment/lifestyle. Research is continuously uncovering the role of epigenetics in a variety of human disorders and fatal diseases.

Expression of Genes: gene expression is the process by which the genetic code - the nucleotide sequence - of a gene is used to direct protein synthesis and produce the structures of the cell. Thus, gene expression involves two main stages:

- *Transcription* – the production of messenger RNA (mRNA) by the enzyme RNA polymerase, and the processing of the resulting mRNA molecule.

- *Translation* – the use of mRNA to direct protein synthesis and the subsequent post-translational processing of the protein molecule.

Frontal Cortex: consists of the two lobes at the front of the head, just behind the forehead, considered the hub of most of the higher brain functions, understanding and most of our behavioural traits. Most long-term planning, emotional regulation, problem-solving, impulse control and motor skills functions is based in this area of the brain.

Genetic Makeup: the genetic makeup of an organism is known as its genotype. The genotype refers to the set of traits found within the cells of living organisms. These traits, known as the genetic code, are passed from one generation to another during cell division and reproduction. 'Genetic makeup' refers to the genes that determine what you look like and what physical characteristics you have; the colour of your eyes, your blood type, hair texture or the structure of your digestive enzymes, etc.

Grey Brain Matter: contains most of the brain's neuronal cell bodies and refers to unmyelinated neurons and other cells of the central nervous system. It is present in the brain, brainstem and cerebellum, and throughout the spinal cord. The grey matter includes regions of the brain involved in muscle control and sensory perception such as seeing and hearing, memory, emotions, speech. For many years it was believed that the human brain is essentially hard-wired, that we are born with a set of cognitive abilities, such as the ability to learn language, which are more or less unalterable for the rest of our lives. However, the discovery of neuroplasticity – our brain's ability to selectively transform itself – refers to our brain's *malleability*, its ability to respond to certain intrinsic or extrinsic stimuli by reorganising its structure, function and connections.

Hippocampus: a brain region of the brain associated primarily with memory. The name hippocampus is derived from the Greek (*hippos*, meaning 'horse' and *kampos*, meaning 'sea monster'); its structure resembles that of a sea horse. The hippocampus, located in the inner (medial) region of the temporal lobe, forms part of the limbic system, which is particularly important in regulating emotional responses. The hippocampus is principally thought to be involved in storing long-term memories and in making those memories resistant to forgetting. However, this is a matter of debate. It is also thought to play an important role in spatial processing and navigation.

Hum: a sound made by producing a wordless tone with the mouth opened or closed, forcing the sound to emerge from the nose usually. Emit a prolonged droning sound like that of the speech sound, often with a melody.

Hunches in the mind: are formed out of our *past experiences and knowledge.* Hunches, often referred to as *intuitions,* or *gut feelings,* don't always lead to good decisions, but are not nearly as flighty a concept as they may seem:

- ❖ "Trust your hunches. They are usually based on facts filed away just below the conscious level." – Dr Joyce Brothers.

❖ "All human knowledge thus begins with intuitions, proceeds thence to concepts and ends with ideas." – Immanuel Kant.

❖ "The intuitive mind is a sacred gift and the rational mind is a faithful servant. We have created a society that honours the servant and has forgotten the gift." – Albert Einstein.

Huntington's disease: a progressive disease of the nervous system marked by tremor, muscular rigidity and slow, imprecise movement, chiefly affecting middle-aged and elderly people. It is associated with degeneration of the basal ganglia of the brain and a deficiency of the neurotransmitter dopamine.

Hypothalamus: its primary function is homeostasis, maintaining the body's status quo, system-wide. A section of the brain responsible for producing many of the body's essential hormones that govern physiological functions such as temperature regulation, thirst, hunger, sleep, mood, sex drive and the release of other hormones within the body. This area of the brain houses the pituitary gland. Although this portion of the brain is small, it is involved in many necessary processes of the body including behavioural, autonomic (involuntary or unconscious) and endocrine functions, such as metabolism, growth and development.

Infinite Intelligence: supposedly the glue that connects all living things with a 'higher intelligence'. It links the senses to the conscious mind and is the inspiration that seems to flow from another place. Whether you believe in God or just in the existence of a 'higher intelligence', its adherents believe *'Infinite Intelligence'* is everywhere in the Universe, and that it comes *from* it to us, and flows back *to* it from us, in a constant ebb and flow.

Insula: an oval region found in each hemisphere of the cerebral cortex, situated within the sylvian fissure, involved in sensation, emotion and autonomic function.

Invigorated: an idea, a concept, philosophy, thing or person that makes you feel fresher, healthier, energetic, driven, focused or inspired.

Limbic brain: a system of the brain containing a group of structures that govern emotions and behaviour. The limbic system, particularly the hippocampus and amygdala, is involved in the formation of long-term memory and is closely associated with the olfactory structures (sense of smell).

MAOA gene: (monoamine oxidase A): Also known as the 'warrior gene', involved in preparing the mind and body for action, the MAOA gene manifests as an aggressive trait that shows more with provocation. Monoamine oxidase A is an enzyme that breaks down important neurotransmitters in the brain, including dopamine, norepinephrine and serotonin. Studies found a link between the low activity form of MAOA and heightened aggression. It cannot be prevented by diet or medication but is controllable, and you can refrain from 'psychotic outbreaks'.

Meditation: a mental practice where an individual trains the mind or induces a mode of consciousness, either to realise some benefit or for the mind to simply acknowledge its content without becoming identified with that content or as an end in itself.

Mind Empowerment: a multi-dimensional social and psychological training process that helps people gain personal development and control over their own lives and communities by acting on issues that they define as important; the concept of empowerment depends upon the idea that power can 'expand our minds', e.g. NLP - the practice of understanding how people can filter and organise their mental maps of the world - thinking, feeling, language and behaviour - to provide a methodology to achieve outstanding performance.

Mindfulness: the psychological process of bringing one's attention to the internal and external experiences occurring in the *present moment*, which can be developed through the practise of meditation and other training. The popularity of mindfulness in the 'West' is generally considered to have been initiated by Jon Kabat-Zinn in the latter part of the 20th Century.

172

Mirror Neuron: a neuron that fires both when an animal acts and when the animal observes the same action performed by another. Thus, the neuron 'mirrors' the behaviour of the other, as though the observer was itself acting. In humans, brain activity consistent with that of mirror neurons has been found in the premotor cortex, the supplementary motor area, the primary somatosensory cortex and the inferior parietal cortex.

Motor Neurons: first identified around 1898, they are nerve cells that conduct impulses to a muscle, gland or other effector, making them either contract or relax. In humans, movement of the articulated internal skeletal structure is enabled by *coordinating* the contractions of the many muscles attached to it. Only the brain is capable of this complex coordination, and electrical signalling is arguably the only means fast enough to deliver its instructions to far-flung muscles. The medium of delivery are electrically excitable cells called neurons.

Its basic structure includes a receptor on one end and a transmitter on the other, connected by an elongated body called the axon, some of which can be 39 inches (1m) long in humans. Chains of nerve cells, end to end, are bundled into nerve fibres, which reach from the brain to the finger muscles and further.

Music Therapy: a technique of complementary medicine that is an established psychological clinical intervention, which is delivered by professionally trained music therapists, to help people of all ages, whose lives have been affected by injury, illness or disability, through supporting their psychological, communicative, emotional, cognitive, physical, and social needs in a skilled manner.

Neurodegenerative Diseases: include Parkinson's, Alzheimer's, and Huntington's. They occur as a result of incurable neurodegenerative processes, resulting in progressive degeneration and death. Research shows many similarities relate these diseases to one another on a sub-cellular level that offers hope for therapeutic advances that could ameliorate many diseases simultaneously.

Neurofibrillary Tangles: intracellular clump of abnormal structures, composed of twisted masses of protein fibres within nerve cells made of insoluble protein, in the brain of patients with Alzheimer's disease.

Neuroplasticity: the brain's ability to reorganise itself by forming new neural connections throughout life. Neuroplasticity allows neurons (nerve cells) in the brain to compensate for injury and disease and to adjust their activities in response to new situations or changes in their environment.

Neuroscience: a multidisciplinary branch of biology that studies the anatomy, biochemistry, molecular biology, physiology, and development of neurons and neural circuits; focusing on the brain and its impact on behaviour and cognitive functions. Neuroscience is not only concerned with the normal functioning of the nervous system, but also what happens when people have neurodevelopmental, psychiatric, or neurological disorders.

Obsessive-Compulsive Disorder (OCD): a condition where a person commonly has obsessive thoughts and compulsive behaviours. Affecting men, women and children, this mental health condition can develop at any age. *Obsession* is an unwanted and unpleasant thought, image, or urge that repeatedly enters the affected person's mind, causing feelings of anxiety, disgust, or unease. *Compulsion* is a repetitive behaviour or mental act that the affected person feels they need to carry out to try to temporarily relieve the unpleasant feelings brought on by the obsessive thought.

Optimistic: positive psychology studies the positive impact that optimism has on mental and physical health. Optimists are seldom sick and live longer than pessimists. A positive outlook on life strengthens the immune system and consequently the body's defences against illness and disease. Optimists have fewer heart attacks, have enhanced responses in dealing with stress and mental illness, and recover from illnesses faster.

Paranormal: Beyond the range of normal experience or scientific explanation.

Parapsychology: the scientific study of interactions between living organisms and their external environment that seems to transcend the known physical laws of nature, which is concerned with the investigation of paranormal and psychic phenomena.

Parkinson's Disease: a progressive neurological condition affecting the brain. Symptoms are caused, in part, by reduced dopamine levels within the brain. Dopamine is a chemical used to transmit messages between brain cells. Brain cells within the region called the *basal ganglia* begin to deteriorate, and dopamine levels start to fall. When levels fall to about 60% of normal, movement symptoms begin to develop. It is not yet known why the cells start to deteriorate. Parkinson's causes both 'motor' and 'non-motor' symptoms.

Motor (or movement) symptoms consist of:

- *Tremor* – involuntary shaking of arms, legs and/or head. It usually affects one side of the body before the other.
- *Rigidity* – stiffness of the limbs.
- *Bradykinesia* – slowness of movement; for example, difficulty turning over in bed or doing up buttons.
- *Postural instability* – impaired postural reflexes; making it difficult to adjust or maintain balance.

- *Non-motor symptoms:* can include depression, anxiety, pain, loss of sense of smell, sleep disturbance, bladder problems, constipation, and fatigue.

Pessimism: is usually seen as is an entrenched negative habit of mind that can have disastrous consequences: depressed mood, resignation to negative experiences, underachievement and even poor physical and mental health. Although, some research seems to indicate that 'defensive pessimism' can result in positive outcomes.

Philanthropy: an altruistic concern for human advancement and welfare, usually manifested by donations of money, property or work to needy persons, by endowment of institutions of learning and hospitals and by generosity to other socially useful purposes.

Phoneme: the smallest meaningful unit of sound in a language. A meaningful sound is one that will change one word into another word. For example, the words cat and fat are two different words, but only one sound is different between the two words – the first sound. That means that the 'k' sound in cat and the 'f' sound in fat are two different morphemes.

Shortly after birth, a baby begins to learn the phonemes of the language used around them. It is part of what they absorb as they learn language. We do not have to teach babies those sounds; their brains are 'hard-wired' to learn them as they interact with people. (It is one of the reasons it's good to talk to babies a lot). As children continue to learn language they aren't consciously aware that words they are learning are made up of separate and very distinct sounds.

Placebo: a substance or other kind of 'treatment' that looks just like a regular treatment or medicine, but it is not. It's actually an *inactive*, inert, treatment, injection, procedure or substance. Typically, the person getting a placebo doesn't know the treatment isn't real but the 'effect' can be real. The term 'Placebo Effect' refers to the helpful effects, a placebo has in relieving symptoms for a short time. It is thought to have something to do with the body's natural chemical ability to relieve pain and certain other symptoms briefly.

Pre-frontal Medial Cortex (PFC): is located in the very front of the brain, just behind the forehead. In charge of abstract thinking and thought analysis, it is also responsible for regulating behaviour. This includes *mediating* conflicting thoughts, making choices between right and wrong and predicting the probable outcomes of actions or events. This brain area also governs social control. The pre-frontal cortex is the brain centre responsible for taking in data through the body's senses and deciding on actions; it is most strongly implicated in human qualities such as consciousness, general intelligence and personality.

Quorum Sensing: the regulation of gene expression in response to fluctuations in cell-population density. Quorum sensing bacteria produce and release chemical signal molecules called auto-inducers that increase in concentration as a function of cell density, which leads to an alteration in gene expressions that regulate a diverse array of physiological activities, including symbiosis, virulence, competence, conjugation, antibiotic production, motility, sporulation and biofilm formation.

Single-Nucleotide Polymorphism: often abbreviated to SNP, is a variation in a single nucleotide that occurs at a specific position in the genome, where each variation is present to some appreciable degree within a population.

Synchronisation: the coordination of events to operate a system in unison. The familiar conductor of an orchestra serves to keep the orchestra in time. Systems operating with all their parts in synchrony are said to be synchronous or in sync; those which are not are asynchronous.

Therapeutic: of or relating to the treating or curing of disease.

Tranquillity: the quality or state of peacefulness, calmness, quietude or serenity.

Velopharyngeal: of or relating to the soft palate and the pharynx.

Ventral Tegmental Area: the origin of dopaminergic neurons of the mesolimbic and mesocortical systems, which project to the nucleus accumbens, amygdala, olfactory tubercle and pre-frontal cortex.

Visualising: by visualising a certain event, situation or an object, you attract it into our life. It is a process similar to daydreaming. For some people, this might look like magic, but there is no magic involved, only the natural process of the power of thoughts and natural mental laws. It is like having a genie at your disposal.

Yoga: an ancient form of exercise focusing on postures to increase strength, flexibility, balance and enhanced breathing, to boost physical and mental wellbeing. There is evidence that regular yoga practice is beneficial for people with high blood pressure, heart disease, aches, pains, depression and stress.

References

1. Byrne, R., 2006. The Secret. 10th ed. UK: Simon and Schuster.

2. Chopra, D. and Tanzi, R., 2014. You Can Transform Your Own Biology [online]. The Chopra Center. Available at: https://chopra.com/articles/you-can-transform-your-own-biology [Accessed 20 March, 2020].

3. Dispenza, J., 2014. You Are The Placebo: Making Your Mind Matter. UK: Hay House, Inc.

4. Doidge, N., 2008. The Brain That Changes Itself. UK: Penguin Books.

5. Goleman, D., 1998. Working with emotional intelligence. 1998. New York and Canada: Bantam.

6. Hamilton, D.R., 2010. How Your Mind Can Heal Your Body? London: Hay House, Inc.

7. Hill, N., 2004. Think and Grow Rich. 1st ed. UK: Vermilion/Edbury Publishing.

8. Lipton, B.H., 2015. The Biology of Belief. 10th ed. New York: Hay House, Inc.

9. Martha, L., 2015. Mindfulness Made Easy. UK: McGraw Hill.

10. Ozaniec, N., 2010. Beat Stress with Meditation: Teach Yourself. 2nd ed. London: Hodder Headline.

11. Sacks, O., 2008, Musicophilia: Tales of Music and the Brain. London: Picador.

12. Schwartz, D., 2015. The Magic of Thinking Big. UK: Simon and Schuster.

13. Shiv, K., 2013. You Can Win. India: Bloomsbury.

14. Usmar, J. and Hibberd, J., 2015. This Book Will Make You Mindful. London: Quercus.

Research Papers Reviewed

1. Banker, L., 2015. The Effectiveness of Music Therapy in Treating Symptoms of Alzheimer's disease. Department of Applied Psychology OPUS.

2. Benioff Childen's Hospital, UCSF, 2012. Treating Neurological Disorders with Music Therapy.

3. Chakravarthi, K., et al., 2015. The Effect of Listening to Music on Human Transcriptome. Peer J.3.

4. Marchard, W.R., 2014. Neural Mechanism of Mindfulness and Meditation: Evidence from Neuroimaging Studies. World Journal of Radiology, 6, 471– 479.

5. Rafal, M., et al., 2014. Effect of Meditation on Cognitive Functions in Context of Aging and Neurodegenerative Diseases. Frontiers in Behavioural Neuroscience 8:17.

6. Alison, M., 2015. Mindfulness and Meditation Effects on Cognition. Frontiers in Behavioural Neuroscience 8.

7. Daniel A. M., 2014. Meditation and Neuro Degenerative Diseases. Annals of the New York Academy of Sciences. ISSN0077- 8923.

8. Bruggen-Rafi. V., Monique, and Roos. R., 2015. The Effect of Music Therapy for Patients with Huntington's disease. Journal of Literature and Art studies, 5, 30-40

9. Wan, Catherine Y., et al., 2010. The Therapeutic Effects of Singing in Neurological Disorders, 27 (4), 287-295.

10. Zeidan, F. Fadel., 2014. The Neurobiology of Mind Fullness Meditation: Chapter 10, 'The Basic Science of Mindfulness'.

Prof. Anees Akhtar

M.Phil. (Microbiology) Author, Journalist, TV and Radio Communicator, Tutor and Mentor

Anees has an MSc in Botany, M.Phil. Microbiology (PAK) and a Post Graduate Diploma in Biotechnology (UK). He works as a Neuroscience, Space Science, Cosmology and Metaphysics Researcher and is a widely respected scholar, thinker, motivational speaker, and seminar leader.

He has delivered many seminars and workshops in universities and institutions in UK and Pakistan. His work in Neuroscience, Metaphysics, Cosmology and Success Philosophy is widely recognised and admired for its lucidity and clarity.

He possesses outstanding ability to transform minds from failure to success and from sickness to good health. His methods of teaching and grounding in his philosophy, are clear, effective and easy to understand and implement.

Dr. Muhammad Nasim Khan

PHD, POSTDOC (USA)

Professor Dr Muhammad Nasim Khan, distinguished Productive Scientist of Pakistan (PSP), former Visiting Professor of St. Cloud State University USA, Chairman of the Department of Biotechnology and Zoology in University of Azad Jammu and Kashmir, Pakistan, is the author of 35 high impact factor international research papers, which produced worthy and novel results in the field of Human Molecular Genetic Disorders.

Dr Khan contributed Bona Fides Research to investigate the eradication of neurodegenerative diseases in underprivileged people from societies by genetic counselling and prenatal diagnosis.

He has rendered 36 years of professional services at University of Azad Jammu and Kashmir, training, supervising, and producing several research scholars at PhD, M.Phil. & MSc levels, who are quite productive and instrumental for their country.

Upon marvellous research accomplishments and academic achievements, Dr Khan has been bestowed upon with numerous Research Productivity Awards from PCST Islamabad and consecutively three times adorned Recognition Shield and Certificates by the President of the state of Azad Jammu and Kashmir and Chancellor of the Universities of AJ&K.

The particular role as co-author of this acclaimed book (Neuroscience of Mind Empowerment) which is a breakthrough in Mind Science, he has been honoured and conferred Multifarious International Awards, including the Book Excellence Award (2019), Independent Press Award (2019) and NYC Big Book Award (2018). The therapeutic ideas given in this book may heal and empower dysfunctional organs and mind in humans.

www.ingramcontent.com/pod-product-compliance
Lightning Source LLC
Chambersburg PA
CBHW060321030426
42336CB00011B/1145